inco
be c

Le

he Greatest Guide to

limming
& Healthy
iving

This is a **GREATEST**GUIDES title

Greatest Guides Limited, Woodstock, Bridge End, Warwick CV34 6PD, United Kingdom

www.greatestguides.com

Series created by Harshad Kotecha

Greatest Guides is committed to a sustainable future for our planet. This book is printed on paper certified by the Forest Stewardship Council.

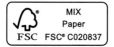

Printed and bound in the United Kingdom

ISBN 978-1-907906-00-8

To my husband Gordon, thanks for being so supportive!

A few words from Wendy …

There are more commercial diets and diet books to choose from than ever before, and each year thousands of people join a gym – yet nearly one in two men and one in three women is overweight. Populations around the world are far heavier than they were fifty years ago. The reasons are simple – we eat more fatty, refined and sugary foods than our parents and grandparents did, and we aren't as physically active in our daily lives.

I've been interested in health and staying slim since I was a teenager. When I gained weight during my teens and early twenties, I lost it by dieting. During my mid-thirties, the pounds crept on again. I did nothing about it, until my late thirties, when I was studying nutrition as part of a health degree. This time I applied what I'd learned and ate a more balanced diet. I also realized my weight gain was linked to eating for reasons other than hunger, so I worked on having a more normal relationship with food. This time the weight came off, and has stayed off.

I firmly believe staying slim, healthy and fit, involves finding a balanced way of eating and living that suits you in the long-term, rather than following a strict diet – a short-term solution that will inevitably fail. It's also about building more activity into your daily life, rather than joining a gym you're unlikely to attend. In this book you'll find tips based on my personal experiences and what I've learned from studying nutrition and health for a number of years.

Contents

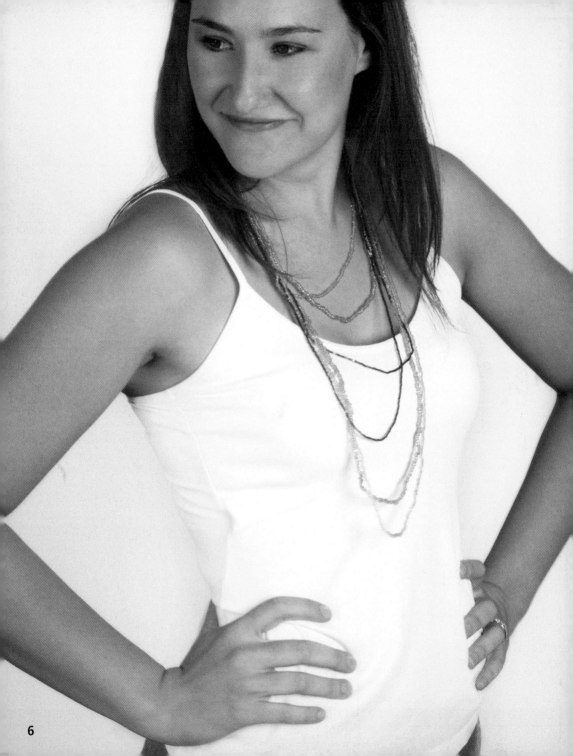

Think Thin

" Dieting is wishful shrinking. "

Anon

Chapter 1
Think Thin

We're constantly bombarded with information about healthy eating. There are more commercial diets to choose from than ever before. Yet, according to the World Health Organization (WHO) 1.6 billion adults around the world were overweight in 2005 and this figure will increase to 2.3 billion by 2015. Clearly, knowing what and how much we should eat in order to be a healthy weight is only part of the story; what and why we eat is also strongly linked to unconscious emotions and past experiences. Many of us indulge in emotional, or comfort eating, to help us deal with negative emotions such as fear, anger, sadness and low self-esteem. Often we turn to foods we learned to associate with comfort during childhood, such as chocolate, potato chips (crisps) and ice cream. This chapter looks at the psychological aspects of weight gain and weight loss, and how to harness the power of your subconscious mind to help you lose weight.

No more excuses!

Go on, be honest! Do you find excuses for being overweight, such as, 'I don't really eat much, it's my metabolism', or, 'I've always been big.' If you're overweight, research shows that you're likely to have a faster metabolism than a slimmer person, because you need more calories to maintain your weight and body's basic functioning. And even if you have always been overweight, you can still lose weight by changing your eating habits and activity levels.

It's in my genes!

'Other members of my family are big,' is another common excuse. Whilst research suggests around one in six people carry the FTO, or so-called 'fat gene', which can make them 3kg (7lbs) heavier than those who don't, this needs to be put into context. Only 30 percent of those with one flawed FTO gene and 70 percent of those with two, are more likely to be overweight. A person carrying seven excess pounds isn't classified as obese. So the majority of people with a weight problem can't blame it on their genes!

What you're more likely to have inherited from your family members are the lifestyle habits that lead to weight gain – i.e. eating a poor diet, overeating and being inactive.

It's my glands

This is another common reason given for being overweight. However, whilst an underactive thyroid (hypothyroidism) is linked to weight gain, it's estimated that only around one in twenty overweight people suffer from it; and even if you are diagnosed with the condition, it is still possible to lose weight with appropriate medication and lifestyle changes.

QUICK T!P

HUNGER PANGS
Another common excuse for not losing weight is 'I'm always hungry'. The answer to this is – you don't have to go hungry to lose weight. If you eat healthy, balanced meals, you're less likely to feel hungry in between. But if you do experience hunger pangs, choose sensible snacks, such as those suggested further on in this book.

It's my age

People do tend to put on weight as they get older, mainly because as they age they usually lose muscle, which makes their metabolism slow down.

However the extra weight is also due to being less physically active than when they were younger, so weight gain in old age isn't inevitable; eating a little less and being more active can help you to maintain a healthy weight.

The real reason why you're overweight

Generally, if you're overweight you're taking in more calories than you're burning off. It's that simple. Facing up to the real reason why you're overweight could be your first step to doing something about it.

Note: Pills that can plump

Several common medicines for conditions such as hay fever, asthma, depression, travel sickness, colds, and insomnia, can lead to weight gain due to increased appetite or fluid retention. Antihistamines, steroids, antidepressants, some of the tablets used to treat type 2 diabetes, and the contraceptive pill, are just some of the medications that can make weight loss more difficult. If you're taking a medication regularly and struggling with losing weight, a discussion with your physician or pharmacist might be a good idea. They might be able to offer an alternative medication that will have less effect on your weight.

Change your unhelpful beliefs about healthy eating

Losing weight usually involves eating more healthily. If you have a negative attitude towards healthy eating you are unlikely to change your eating habits. Below are some common unhelpful beliefs about healthy eating. Try replacing them with the more realistic ones that follow.

Unhelpful belief: Eating healthily costs a lot more.

Reality: Eating healthily can save you money, because fruit, vegetables, legumes and whole grains cost less than meat, takeaways and ready meals.

Unhelpful belief: Healthy food doesn't taste nice.

Reality: Healthy food can taste good, especially if you make lower fat and low sugar versions of your favorite dishes. Buy a healthy cookery book.

Unhelpful belief: Healthy foods don't fill you up.

Reality: Baked (jacket) potatoes, brown rice, wholewheat pasta, beans, peas and lentils are extremely filling and healthy, so long as you don't add lots of fats e.g. butter, margarine or sauces.

Unhelpful belief: I'm too tired to cook a healthy meal when I come home from work.

Reality: Healthy meals can be prepared or even cooked in advance and stored in the fridge or freezer. See No time to cook? in Chapter 3.

Great expectations!

Some people hold the mistaken belief that if they lose weight, their lives will be perfect. They attach all kinds of attributes to slimness, such as confidence, success and attractiveness. Consequently they fear being slim. What if they don't live up to their own or other's expectations? Being overweight becomes a way of avoiding having to be this perfect person with a perfect life.

For others, the opposite may be true – they lose weight because of their belief that their lives will be perfect once they become slim. But, once they lose weight, they realize this isn't the case. Disillusioned, many then start to comfort eat, and consequently regain the weight they lost, and more.

Weight loss may improve your health and boost confidence, but you will still be the same person, with your own unique personality and traits. Changing your shape will not magically change your life, it will simply change your shape!

Once you've accepted this fact, you may find it easier to lose excess pounds, because you'll no longer have unrealistic expectations of yourself, and what your life will be like once you become thin.

Are You Ready To Slim?

You'll only change your eating habits when you're ready. That may sound obvious, but it's surprising how many people are aware that they should lose weight, but do nothing about it. Research suggests this is because most people go through a cycle of stages before they make permanent behavior changes, and will only be successful if they progress to the stage where they're ready to commit to making the necessary changes.

Psychologists Prochaska and DiClemente identified six stages in the cycle – Pre-contemplation, Contemplation, Preparation, Action, Maintenance and Relapse.

Pre-contemplation – This is the stage where you are either unaware of the need to lose weight, or simply have no desire to lose weight.

Contemplation – At this stage you are becoming aware of the need or desire to change your habits and are seriously thinking about doing so. You are likely to have a reason for this change of attitude. Perhaps you're concerned about your health, or maybe you want to improve your appearance. You may start looking at what you need to do to lose weight, i.e. make lifestyle changes, in terms of what and how much you eat and how much exercise you take. But you're not quite ready to make these changes.

Preparation – You've decided to take action. You're beginning to make serious plans to help you achieve your goal, such as identifying your target weight, the date you want to reach it by and how you intend to achieve it.

Action – This is the point where you are ready to take active steps to change your lifestyle. You are now making the changes necessary to bring about weight loss. Your level of motivation is likely to be high and you find it easy to stick to your new eating and activity habits.

Maintenance – This is the hardest part of changing your lifestyle, because the initial enthusiasm might have worn off. Perhaps people are no longer complimenting you on your new shape. Old patterns of comfort eating and overindulging in the wrong types of foods may seem tempting. This is the time when you may need support and encouragement from family and friends. It might help if you revisit the reasons why you wanted to lose weight in the first place and remind yourself of your achievements. Identify situations where you're tempted to overeat and plan strategies to help you resist. Reward yourself with non-food items such as a new perfume, or new clothes.

Relapse – You've returned to your old habits! The key to dealing with this stage is not to panic. Accept that it happens to most people. Then return to the contemplation stage and begin the cycle again. Evidence suggests many people go through the process of change three or more times, before finally leaving behind the lifestyle that made them overweight. The important point to remember is that becoming slimmer and healthier isn't about sticking to a rigid diet. It's more about making lifestyle changes on a long-term basis. If you occasionally overeat it shouldn't lead to weight gain, providing you stick to healthy habits most of the time.

Where are you in the cycle?

Identifying where you are in the cycle can be really helpful, as it will help you decide what your next step should be. If you haven't started trying to lose weight, but you're obviously thinking about it, because you're reading this book, then you're at the contemplation stage. The next step for you is preparation. This is a good time to keep a food diary to identify your eating patterns. You could then make an action plan, setting out your goal and the steps you need to take to achieve it, perhaps incorporating some of the weight loss tips outlined in this book that appeal to you. Then take action by following your action plan. If you've lost weight in the past and then regained it, you're at the relapse stage. It's important that you don't give up, but find ways that suit you to eat less and be more active. This book offers you lots of ideas on how to do this.

What's your motivation?

Losing weight can be difficult, especially initially. So when you're finding sticking to your new eating habits tough, identifying why you want to slim and focussing on the rewards you'll enjoy, can help you to stay on the straight and narrow. For example, your motivation might be that you want to slip into that little black dress, or you want to look good on the beach, or that you simply want to feel better. Focussing regularly on the long-term pleasure you'll gain from achieving your weight loss goal, can help you to resist the short-term pleasures of overeating.

Self-talk and size

Self-talk is a term used to describe the ongoing conversation we have with ourselves. If your self-talk is negative as in 'I'll never lose weight. I'm fat and I can't change,' it'll perpetuate a negative self-image, which your actions will reflect, probably in the form of overeating. Equally, if you make sure your self-talk is constructive, by creating positive affirmations using the methods outlined overleaf, you will find yourself acting in ways that support this positive view of yourself.

Affirm and slim

An affirmation is a positive statement you make about yourself. It needs to be personal, so use the word 'I'. It must be positive, so state what you want to achieve, not what you don't. It's also more effective if you write it as though it's happening now. So a good weight loss affirmation would incorporate all of these points. For example, 'I am slim and healthy', rather than 'I will not be overweight and unfit'. This imprints in your subconscious mind a clear image of the result you want to achieve, as though you've already achieved it.

Attaching positive emotions to your goal will make it seem more real and achievable. You'll also see results more quickly, e.g. 'I am slim, healthy, happy and energetic'.

To fix your affirmation in your subconscious mind, first read it. Next, close your eyes and see the image your words conjure up. Picture yourself experiencing your goal in detail. Visualize yourself slim. Imagine the clothes you'll wear. Feel the emotions you've attached to your goal. Hear the words your family and friends will use to compliment you on your appearance. Reading, picturing, feeling and hearing your affirmation has a powerful effect on your subconscious mind. Do this on a daily basis and you should quickly find yourself adopting behaviors to support this new image you have of yourself i.e. healthy habits, such as eating a balanced diet and being more active.

Seeing is believing

Remember, your subconscious mind can't tell the difference between what's happened in reality, and what's occurred in your imagination. If you regularly visualize yourself slim, your subconscious mind will believe you're already slim and you'll find yourself acting like a slim person.

Set specific and realistic targets

Set yourself a specific and realistic target such as 'I will lose 450g (1lb) per week'.

You're more likely to be successful than if you simply state 'I want to lose weight', or if you set yourself unrealistic goals such as 'I will lose 6.5kg (1 stone) in a month'.

Identify your eating patterns

Keep a food and drink diary for a week, recording not only when you ate, but also how hungry you were, what and how much you ate, where, who with, and how you felt at the time e.g. stressed, happy, sad, angry, upset. This will help you identify the eating patterns that are sabotaging your efforts to lose weight. For example, eating when you're stressed or bored, rather than hungry. You can then plan strategies to overcome them.

Sample Food Diary

Date/time	Hunger level	Food eaten/ drinks	Where & who with	Feelings

Mind mindless eating

It's important that you record everything you eat. If you habitually eat the kids' or your partner's leftovers without thinking, you need to include it in your diary. If you regularly taste-test while you cook – that counts too! Eating just 100 calories a day more than you need, can lead to a 10lb weight gain in a year. Make it a rule to throw your family's leftovers away and stop taste-testing in the kitchen; this could help you lose pounds!

Manage stress

Research shows that long-term stress leads to over-production of the stress hormones adrenaline and cortisol. Eating sugary and fatty foods seems to counteract their effects by inducing feelings of calm. If you tend to overeat or binge on junk foods when stressed, try to find other ways to relax. For example, practise deep breathing, exercise, listen to music, or drink chamomile tea. After a stressful day at work, enjoy a long relaxing soak in the bath, rather than heading straight for the food cupboard. Do whatever works for you. If you're stressed because of a problem, try to find a solution, or talk it through with someone you trust, rather than turning to food. For more ideas on stress relief see Chapter 9 – Stress Busters.

Beat boredom

If you tend to eat when bored, plan ways to beat boredom that don't involve food. Read that new novel you've been meaning to read. Catch up with the friend you haven't seen for ages. Find a new interest that excites you. That way you'll 'eat to live' rather than 'live to eat'.

Feel rather than 'eat' emotions

If you comfort eat to suppress emotions such as anger, or hurt, explore ways to express and deal with your feelings, such as talking them through with an appropriate person, or writing them down. Identify any underlying issues or problems and seek solutions, so that you can treat food as fuel for your body, rather than an escape from your emotions. Food may provide a temporary distraction or comfort, but the emotions or problems you're trying to distance yourself from will still be there, probably with the added problem of weight gain.

So next time you find yourself dipping into the cookie (biscuit) tin ask yourself 'Am I hungry for food, or is something bothering me?'

Swap bad habits for good ones

A habit is something you do several times until it becomes ingrained in your patterns of behavior and you can do it almost without thinking. What you eat, and how often, is largely based on habits – often formed during childhood. So to lose weight you need to replace bad eating habits with good ones. Once you have carried out the new behavior several times, it too becomes a habit and therefore easier to stick to.

QUICK T!P
FOLLOW THE 80:20 RULE
Don't beat yourself up if you overindulge sometimes. Evidence suggests that if you eat healthily 80 percent of the time, you needn't worry about the other 20 percent.

Meal planner

Planning your meals in advance makes it less likely that you'll grab a takeaway, or fill up on junk food. Take healthy snacks such as nuts, seeds, fruit, or chopped raw vegetables, to work with you, so that you're less likely to be tempted by the cookie (biscuit) tin. Make your own packed lunch, or find a sandwich shop that offers wholemeal bread and healthy fillings. If you must eat fast-food, think about how you can make it healthier, before you order (see also pages 64–66).

To weigh, or not to weigh?

Regular weighing can help weight loss and maintenance by boosting morale and acting as an early warning system. But if you find you've gained weight it can depress and demotivate. It's important to take a long-term view and remember that hormonal fluctuations in women, and water retention, can account for several extra pounds; so long as your weight is generally going down, or has stabilised at a healthy level, the occasional hiccup doesn't matter. Strength training can increase weight, because muscle weighs more than fat – here it's better to monitor your progress with a tape measure, or by how your clothes fit.

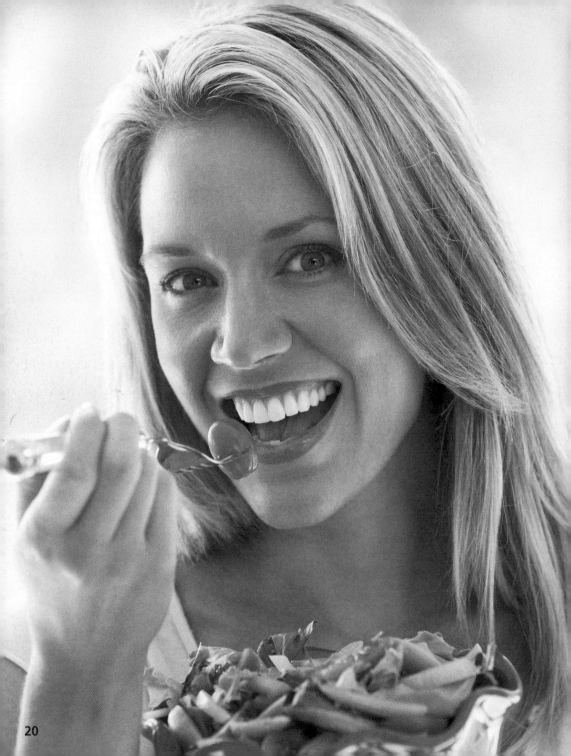

Eat Less

“ Enough is as good as a feast. ”

Anon

Chapter 2
Eat Less

To lose weight we need to take in fewer calories than we burn off. The best way to do this is to eat a healthy, balanced diet on a long-term basis, rather than following fad diets on a short-term basis. Such diets tend to deprive you of your favorite foods, making you more likely to want to eat them; inevitably you will eventually give in to your cravings – and probably end up overindulging in the 'forbidden' foods. I believe it's far better to continue to eat these foods, but in smaller amounts, as part of a balanced diet. However, it's still possible to gain weight whilst eating a healthy diet – if you eat more food than your body needs. So this section suggests dietary and behavioral changes to help you cut down on the amount of food you eat, without having to count calories, or stick to a strict diet regime.

Eating less is difficult because we live in an environment where food, particularly fast and convenience foods, is available 24 hours a day. It's easier than ever to eat too much generally, but particularly foods that are high in fat and sugar and low in nutritional value. It's very easy to eat, whenever we feel the urge. Also our increasingly hectic lifestyles mean that mealtimes are often rushed, or we eat 'on the hoof' – habits than can lead to us eating more food than we actually need. To help you beat this, I've suggested strategies that will make it harder for you to overeat.

Introduce new behaviors gradually, perhaps only one at a time. Even if you only adopt one change, it could be enough to alter your eating habits for life and to enable you to lose weight and keep it off permanently.

Body Mass Indicator

Before you make any changes to your eating habits, check whether you're overweight. The current most popular method is to work out your Body Mass Indicator (BMI).

To calculate your BMI, multiply your height in meters by your height in meters. Then divide your weight in kilograms by this figure. For example, if you were 1.6m (5ft 3in) tall and weighed 65kg (10st) you would work it out like this:

1.6 meters x 1.6 meters = 2.56

BMI = 65 divided by 2.56 = 25.39

BMI Ratings

Less than 18.5 – underweight

18.5 – 24.9 – healthy weight

25.0 – 29.9 – overweight

30.0 – 39.9 – obese

40.0 and above – morbid obesity

A BMI of 25.39 would indicate the need to lose a little weight. But remember your BMI is only a guide. A muscular person with little fat would still have a high BMI, as it measures weight, rather than fat, in relation to height.

QUICK T!P

BE WAIST WISE

Another indicator that you need to lose weight is your waist size. Carrying too much fat around your middle increases you risk of serious health problems such as heart disease, high blood pressure, stroke, diabetes and certain cancers. A waist size of 80cm (32 inches) for a woman and 94cm (37 inches) for a man, indicates increased risk. For women, an 88cm (35 inches) or above, and for men a 102cm (40 inches) or above waist, means your risk of ill-health is high. This is because fat cells around the tummy release chemicals that can raise blood pressure and cholesterol levels, as well as affect how the body uses insulin. To reduce your waist size you need to combine healthy eating with being more active.

Chop or change!

Keep a food diary as outlined in the Think Thin section. Check what and how much you're eating. Most people underestimate how much they actually eat and find this exercise an eye-opener. Next decide what you could cut down on, or omit altogether – for example one cookie (biscuit) instead of two, no cream in your coffee, no mid-afternoon snack. Look for lower-fat alternatives to your favorite foods, so that you eat less saturated fat. For example oven fries (chips) instead of fried, low-fat, rather than creamy yogurt, Twiglets, rather than potato chips (crisps). For more food swap ideas, see Chapter 3 Eat More Healthily. Note: Be aware that low fat versions of cookies (biscuits) and cakes etc tend to contain more sugar.

QUICK T!P

CUT 100

Cutting around 100 calories from your daily intake will enable you to lose around 4.5kg (10lb) in a year. That could mean simply cutting out one cookie (biscuit) a day, or six teaspoons of sugar, or one packet of potato chips (crisps). A small change with a big result!

Less is more!

When you reduce your food intake, you will probably find that you enjoy your food far more. When you overeat, you go beyond the point when eating is pleasurable.

Go for low GI ...

The Glycemic Index (GI) indicates the rate at which a food raises the level of sugar in the blood. Carbohydrates with a high GI include refined foods such as white bread, pastries, sugary drinks and candy, which are easily converted into glucose and cause your blood sugar to rise rapidly.

Carbohydrates with a low GI, such as multigrain bread, oatmeal (porridge), sweet potatoes, pasta, and basmati or brown rice, take longer to digest and cause your blood glucose to rise slowly, making you feel full longer and therefore eat less. Low GI foods also reduce the risk of type 2 diabetes.

For a low GI diet, replace all refined carbohydrates such as white bread, cookies (biscuits), pastries and sweets, with whole grains. Eat lots of fruit and vegetables, low fat dairy products, such as yogurt, low fat (1 percent fat) milk, low fat cheese and yogurt, and small amounts of nuts, fish and lean meat. Leave the skins on potatoes, to keep their GI low – eating potatoes without the skin enables the glucose to be digested more quickly. New potatoes boiled in their skins have the lowest GI.

Sticking to these types of foods also helps to dispel excess fat around the stomach, which is believed to increase the risk of heart disease, high blood pressure and type 2 diabetes.

... and high satiety

Satiety is the term used to describe the feeling of fullness and satisfaction you experience after eating. The satiety index has been devised to rate foods in terms of their ability to satisfy hunger. The longer a food makes you feel full, the higher its rating. Research suggests that high-volume, low-calorie foods make you feel content more quickly and for longer, so that you're less likely to overeat. Foods with a high water content, such as fruit, vegetables and fish, fit into this category.

If you eat high-calorie low-volume foods, such as full-fat cheese, or chocolate, you're likely to ingest a lot more calories before your brain signals to you that you are full. For example, if you ate grapes in their dried form – as raisins, you would take in 100 calories after eating only one quarter of a cup, but you could eat a cup full of fresh grapes and still only consume 100 calories. Instead of the full-fat cheese or chocolate, you could eat higher-volume lower-calorie foods like cottage cheese, or chocolate mousse. So if you want to lose weight, aim at eating foods with lots of bulk, but low in calories. Foods with a high satiety score include baked potatoes, fish, oatmeal (porridge), oranges, apples, wholewheat pasta, steak, grapes and unsweetened popcorn.

Loaded

Another term you may come across is Glycemic Load (GL). It's possible for a food to have a high GI, but a low GL. Confused? In a nutshell, GL is a measure of how much a 'normal' portion of a particular food affects blood sugar. The Glycemic Index is based on a portion containing 50g of carbohydrate, which could be quite a large amount. So, it's possible for a high GI food to have a low GL. For example, ice cream has a high GI, but a low GL – when you eat just a couple of scoops. Basically, this means you can eat foods like ice cream in small amounts, without affecting your blood sugar too much. Again the message is, keep refined sugary and starchy foods to a minimum!

QUICK T!P

EAT BREAKFAST
Studies show that people who eat breakfast tend to eat less during the day and as a result are usually slimmer. Choose low GI foods such as wholegrain bread or oatmeal (porridge). Adding protein in the form of skim, reduced-fat or low-fat (1 percent fat) milk, or eggs, will keep your blood sugar steady.

Protein power

Ensuring you eat protein foods such as meat, fish, eggs and cheese at each meal can help you to eat less, and burn more calories and fat.

Protein makes you feel fuller for longer, because it slows down the rate at which the body digests food. When protein is eaten with carbohydrates, glucose is released more slowly into the bloodstream. Research showed that people whose diet was about one third protein ate, on average, 441 calories less each day than those whose diet contained around one sixth protein.

Protein also seems to boost the metabolism for up to three hours, so you burn more calories. It's claimed that the body burns around one third of the calories from protein foods whilst processing them. It also encourages the body to burn fat for energy. But beware, animal proteins are high in saturated fats, so go for low-fat dairy foods and lean meats.

Go to work on an egg!

It seems this famous advert slogan encouraging us to eat eggs offered good advice. A study at Louisiana State University in the U.S. showed that women who ate two eggs and toast at breakfast felt so full and satisfied, they ate nearly 300 fewer calories each day, than women who ate bagels and cream cheese. A later study by the same researchers compared the weight loss of two groups of women on low-fat diets. One group ate two eggs for breakfast, whilst the other ate a bagel containing roughly the same number of calories. After eight weeks the women who ate eggs for breakfast had lost 65 percent more weight and more inches from their waistline, than those who ate bagels.

Sip soup

Non-creamy soups such as vegetable, carrot and coriander, or tomato and basil are nutritious, low in calories and filling. A study showed that eating chicken and vegetable soup keeps you full for one hour longer than if you drink water followed by a meal of chicken and vegetables.

Eat your favorite foods

Basing your diet on foods you really enjoy, rather than on foods you feel you should eat, means you're less likely to feel deprived and go on an eating binge. It's human nature to want what you think you can't have! However, you may need to adapt your favorite recipes to make them lower in fat and sugar. Aim at developing a taste for healthier foods, so that you can still satisfy your palate, whilst managing your weight.

Chew gum

Chewing gum between meals has been shown to reduce appetite and decrease food intake at mealtimes by around a third. Choose sugar-free for fewer calories and better dental health.

QUICK T!P

DON'T SHOP ON AN EMPTY STOMACH!
Eat before you go food shopping. Studies show that when you shop on an empty stomach you're more likely to buy fatty, sugary foods.

Shopping list

Writing a shopping list before you go, and sticking to it, also helps to ensure you buy only the foods you really need. Set yourself a time limit – the less time you spend at the supermarket the less likely you are to buy things that aren't on your list.

Small is beautiful

Research reveals that people eat up to forty-five percent more food when it's in a large pack. In one study, people with a large box containing 400g (1lb) of spaghetti ate up to a third more than another group, who were given a small box containing the same amount of spaghetti. So go for foods in smaller packs at the supermarket.

Self-checkout

Research suggests that using the self-checkout till at your supermarket makes you 50 percent less likely to buy foods on impulse.

QUICK T!P
MAKE MEALTIMES AN OCCASION
Sit at the table. Set the table properly and add little touches like fresh napkins, or flowers, to make it look inviting. Play relaxing music. If you make meal times more of an occasion you'll be less likely to bolt your food and overeat.

Make snacking an occasion too

If you make it a rule to eat snacks from a plate at the table too, you'll be less likely to snack on impulse, because it'll require more effort than simply grabbing food and eating it.

Out of sight, out of mind

When food is easy to see and easy to access, we tend to overeat. In a recent trial, secretaries given bowls of chocolates ate half as many when they were placed six feet away, as opposed to when they were placed on their desks. Putting them in a drawer cut the number of chocolates eaten by a third.

So if you want to reduce the number of treats you eat, make sure you place them out of reach, or out of sight. If they're out of reach, you're more likely to think twice about whether you really want them. If they're out of sight you're much less likely to overindulge, because when food is in constant view we tend to think about it more. Thinking about food is often a cue to eat.

Drink more water

Drink more water – it'll fill you up and prevent you mistaking thirst for hunger.

Don't eat ...

- Because it's a meal time

- Because you're starting a diet tomorrow

- Because other people are eating

- Because something is 'eating' you

- Because you've worked hard and you deserve it

- Or any of the other reasons you eat when you're not hungry

Eat ...

Only when you're hungry, and stop when you're full. When you eat only in response to stomach (physiological) hunger, rather than mouth (psychological) hunger, you're eating in keeping with your body's needs, rather than your emotional ones. If you're normally an emotional eater, this means you'll be eating less.

Recognize real hunger

Recognize how your body signals when it's hungry. For most people, hunger manifests itself with contractions in the stomach, but some feel it in the chest or throat. You may experience similar feelings when your appetite is stimulated by the thought, sight, or smell of food. However these sensations are usually temporary, whereas real hunger doesn't fade. Generally, if you have to ask yourself 'Am I hungry?', you're probably not!

Rate your hunger

Reduce the likelihood of overeating by rating how hungry you are before you eat. Try measuring your hunger on a scale of 1 to 4, with 1 signifying you're full, 2 signifying you're peckish, 3 signifying you're hungry and 4 signifying you're ravenous. This can help you to determine how much food you need. For example, if you rate your hunger as a 2, perhaps a smaller plate of food, or a snack, rather than a full meal, will do. If you wait until your hunger rating is 4, you're more likely to crave sweet, starchy foods to give your lowered blood sugar an instant boost, so try to eat when your rating is no more than 3.

Hungry for what?

Your appetite is there not just to tell you when you're hungry, but also what kind of food your body needs – if you listen to it. Your individual nutritional requirements are dependent on many things, including your age, gender and activity levels. For instance, if you've been physically active all day, you're likely to crave more starchy, energy-producing foods, than if you'd just sat in a chair. If you eat what your body is hungry for, you'll probably find you'll be satisfied with less food than if you just eat whatever is to hand.

Heat up

Turn down the air-conditioning at the office, and at home, during hot weather and you should find your appetite decreases.

QUICK T!P
FEMALES NEED LESS FOOD
If you're a woman, remember that in general women need around 500 calories fewer than men, so make sure you serve yourself smaller portions – about a fifth less than your partner's.

Portion control

To maintain a healthy weight, it's vital that you control your portion sizes. Even if you eat healthy foods, if you eat too much of them you'll gain weight.

An easy guide:

- Carbohydrate foods such as pasta, potatoes and rice: 2 handfuls

- Vegetables/salad: 2 handfuls

- Protein foods such as meat, cheese, eggs and fish: 1 handful

- Nuts – 1 small handful

- Fats and oils – 15ml (1 tablespoon) or less

Use a smaller plate

Evidence suggests that the bigger the portion size, the more people will eat; the 'supersizing' of fast food meals is one of the factors blamed for the rise in obesity. Eating from a smaller plate automatically cuts your portion sizes and the sight of an empty plate will trick your brain into thinking that you are full.

Slow down!

If you eat quickly, you can end up eating a lot more food than you need, before your brain realizes you are full. So try to eat slowly and focus on each mouthful. Putting your knife and fork down whilst you chew your food will help you to eat more slowly. Savor the smell, taste and texture of your food. You'll enjoy it more and find it easier to recognise when you've eaten enough, because your body will have time to release leptin, the hormone that signals satisfaction. You'll probably notice that you enjoy your food less as you fill up. This is your body's way of signalling that you've eaten enough. Aim to stop eating when this happens.

Chew it over

An American study showed that people who chewed their food well tended to eat around 70 calories less at each meal and still felt full an hour later. Aim at chewing each mouthful of food at least twenty times.

Conscious eating

When you're tempted to overeat, stop and ask yourself 'Do I really want this food, or am I just eating it because it's there?' Then make a choice whether or not to eat some, or all of the food. This puts you in control, rather than the food.

Avoid distractions

Don't watch TV or read whilst you're eating. By avoiding distractions and giving your food your full attention, you'll probably find that you eat less.

Tune in to your taste buds

When you start eating, focus on the flavor of your food. Does it taste good? It's easy to eat a plateful of food without really tasting it. When you take the time to taste what you're eating, you may decide it's not all that nice and choose not to eat it.

Avoid 'empty plate syndrome'

As a child you may have been encouraged to clear your plate and told it was wasteful not to. Remember, your hunger should determine how much you eat, not the portion size. Practise leaving food on your plate until you feel comfortable with it. If it makes you feel any better, feed your leftovers to the birds!

Watch a slim person eat

You can learn a lot about how to have a normal relationship with food by watching how a slim person, who isn't dieting, eats. They are likely to feel totally at ease with food and their body and find it hard to understand why some people have problems with eating and excess weight. You'll probably notice that he or she will only eat when they are hungry and is very selective about what they eat. They are likely to savor each mouthful of food and stop eating as soon as they start to feel full. They probably won't have a problem with leaving food on the plate.

Take a break

It can take fifteen to twenty minutes for your brain to register that your stomach is full. So if you pause for a few minutes before reaching for that second helping or dessert, you may find you're no longer hungry and can do without.

Eat less in company

Research shows that people eat around a third more food when they eat with another person, as opposed to eating alone. Eat with three and you're likely to eat three quarters more. Eat with a group of seven or more people and you could eat up to 90 percent more. If you're eating at home you're likely to continue eating until everyone has finished, thus possibly eating more than you need to. When eating out we tend to want to prolong the whole eating and social experience, so we're more likely to order a dessert, even if we're full.

To counteract the tendency to eat more in company, aim to be the last person to start eating and the slowest eater. Engaging in conversation is a good ploy – it's difficult to talk and eat at the same time!

Beat buffet binging

It's easy to overeat at buffets – many people ignore their body's 'full-up' signals when faced with a vast array of foods. This is because when we eat only one or two foods, we soon become tired of the taste. If we select lots of different foods and tastes, our tastebuds are stimulated each time and we're more likely to eat too much. Try the following strategies to beat buffet binging:

- Visit the buffet table only once

- Avoid too much pastry

- Fill your plate with mainly protein foods such as chicken – minus the skin – other lean meats, carbohydrate such as bread or rice and plenty of salad

- If you eat dessert, make it a small portion

- Be selective. Only choose foods you enjoy

- Eat slowly and focus on your food, as well as the conversation

- Talking is a good tactic to prevent you from eating too quickly!

- Over-indulging in alcohol can lead to overeating, because it stimulates the appetite and weakens resolve, so alternate alcoholic drinks with non-alcoholic ones

Learn to say 'no'

When you're a guest at someone's home, or attending a function, don't allow yourself to be pressured into eating food out of politeness. When you feel you've eaten enough, or when you're just not hungry, don't be afraid to compliment your host on their delicious food, but state firmly that you just can't eat any more, or you're not hungry.

Do something different

There's evidence that changing your routine by doing something different every day can lead to weight loss. In a study, people following this advice lost an average of nearly 1.5kg (3lbs) a month, without consciously changing their eating or exercise habits. It seems this works because doing new and interesting things forces you to break the old habits which have prevented you from losing weight. One woman found that by breaking her routine of sitting in front of the TV each night, she started to do things she'd been putting off doing, such as clearing the clutter in her home. She went on to take up new interests, and as a side-effect she lost weight. It appears that as people gain more fulfillment in their lives, their weight drops.

You're also less likely to focus on food and eat just for the sake of it. One woman described herself as being less interested in food and more interested in achieving more in her life.

So, if you've thought about trying salsa-dancing or rock-climbing, or even just listening to another radio station, or reading a different newspaper, give it a go – you've nothing to lose but excess weight!

Clean your teeth

Try cleaning your teeth after your evening meal. The fresh, minty taste should make you feel less inclined to snack on sweet foods afterwards.

Sleep and slim

Too little sleep has been shown to affect hormones and metabolism, making overeating and weight gain more likely.

Recent research showed that people who don't get enough sleep eat nearly half as much more than those who do. A hormone called leptin regulates how much we eat by giving the signal of fullness when we've eaten enough. Ghrelin is a hormone which increases hunger – especially for high carbohydrate foods.

People who sleep poorly have been found to have lower levels of leptin, and higher levels of ghrelin, and as a result are more likely to overeat. If you feel that lack of sleep may be contributing to your weight problem, start taking steps now to ensure you get more sleep and you could find yourself eating less and losing weight. Even an extra twenty minutes has been shown to bring about weight loss. See Chapter 10 – Sleep Tight for tips to help you sleep soundly.

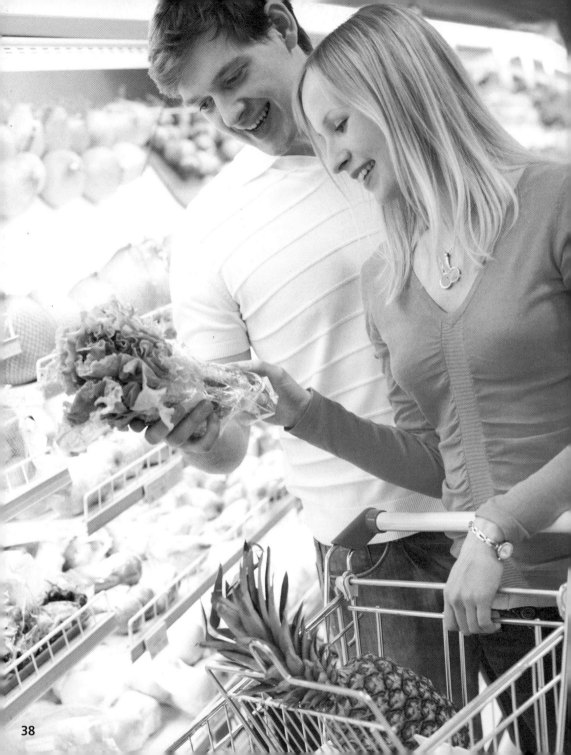

Eat More Healthily

" Food is an important part of a balanced diet. "

Fran Lebowitz

Chapter 3
Eat More Healthily

Being overweight is a risk factor for several health problems. These include high blood pressure, coronary heart disease, stroke, some cancers, type 2 diabetes, osteoarthritis, liver disease and fertility problems. Experts warn that unless obesity rates are reduced, many will die up to nine years earlier than they need to, or have an old age blighted by poor health.

So it's generally accepted that if you want to live a long and healthy life, you need to maintain a healthy weight. If you want to lose weight, it's best to avoid fad diets. Many such diets, including some of the commercial ones, are nutritionally unbalanced and, in the long-term, can lead to weight gain. This is mainly because many of them are so restrictive, it's impossible to stick to them for any length of time. They may bring about weight loss, but as soon as the dieter reverts to 'normal' eating, weight is regained. Often the dieter ends up heavier, because a low-calorie diet will encourage the body to go into 'starvation mode', which means that the metabolism slows down. The body then needs fewer calories, so when more are consumed, they're stored as fat.

Yo-yo dieting – where a person loses weight, regains it and then goes on to lose it again, has been shown to endanger health, because it damages vital organs such as the heart, liver and kidneys and raises the risk of stroke, diabetes and heart disease. It may sound boring, but the secret of healthy, long-lasting weight management is a healthy, balanced diet, along with regular physical activity. Not only is this more effective, it's also cheaper – the cost of attending commercial diet classes can often mean that the only pounds you lose are the ones in your purse or wallet!

Current healthy eating guidelines suggest that around a third of your diet should consist of carbohydrates such as bread, cereal and potatoes and that these should be wholegrain where possible. Fruit and vegetables should make up another third of your diet. The remaining third should be shared roughly equally between dairy and protein foods and a smaller amount of fatty, or sugary foods. Remember though that these are just guidelines and that your individual needs will vary slightly according to your metabolism, how active you are etc. Healthy eating is about getting the balance right. You can still eat fatty and sugary foods – so long as you view them as a treat and eat them sparingly. Eating too many refined and sugary foods has been linked to raised blood sugar levels, which can lead to diabetes, obesity, high blood pressure, heart disease and stroke. But when only your favorite high-calorie treat will do – indulge in a small amount. This is better than trying to stick to an impossibly strict diet whilst craving a food you're not 'allowed'. Eventually you're likely to give in to the craving and go on an eating 'binge', or just abandon the diet. Following a balanced diet helps you to have a more normal relationship with food, rather than an all or nothing 'diet or no-diet' approach.

This chapter offers suggestions to help you follow these guidelines, control your weight and dramatically improve your health, without having to stick to a restrictive diet, or spend a fortune on special diet foods.

QUICK T!P

PERFECT PLATE
For an easy way to ensure a balanced meal, fill roughly one third of your plate with vegetables and/or fruit, a third with carbohydrates and add a handful of a high-protein food.

Feeling fruity?

Eating more fruit and vegetables is probably the easiest way to improve your long-term health and lose weight. Fruit and vegetables generally contain various vitamins, minerals and phytochemicals (plant chemicals), which offer numerous benefits to health, including helping to prevent heart disease and certain cancers. Studies have shown that people who lose weight tend to keep it off, if they base their meals around fruit and vegetables, probably because they provide bulk and a feeling of fullness, leaving less room for sugary, fatty foods. Current recommendations are that we should eat at least five portions of fruit and vegetables a day.

Eat a rainbow

To benefit from a wide range of phytonutrients, make sure you eat fruit and vegetables across the spectrum of colors. These pigments indicate the compounds contained in the plant. Each compound offers various disease-preventing properties. The red color of tomatoes comes from lycopene. Anthocyanins give fruits such as strawberries, cherries, blueberries, plums and grapes their red, blue or purple hues. The orange pigment in carrots is beta-carotene. The yellow pigment in sweetcorn is lutein. Read more about them in Chapter 4 – Superfoods.

What's a portion?

All fruit and vegetables, including fresh, frozen, canned, dried, and pure juices, count. But no matter how much juice you drink, it only counts as one portion, because it doesn't contain all of the fiber of the whole fruit. Also, the sugars are more concentrated and can cause damage to teeth. Potatoes and yams are starchy and are classed as carbohydrates, rather than vegetables because we tend to eat them as a carbohydrate food; sweet potatoes, parsnips, swedes and turnips do count as vegetables, because they are usually eaten as a vegetable along with another carbohydrate food. Pulses such as beans, lentils and peas only count as one portion, whatever amount you eat, because like potatoes, they're quite starchy and don't contain all of the vitamins and antioxidants that fruit and vegetables do.

The World Health Organization recommends that we eat at least 400g (1lb) of fruit and vegetables daily to obtain the nutrients we need for good health. It was decided that the easiest way to achieve this was by eating at least five 80g (2½oz) portions daily. A portion translates roughly into:

- One piece of medium-sized fruit such as an apple, banana, orange, pear, or peach

- A slice of large fruit, for example melon, mango or pineapple

- A cupful of grapes, cherries, or berries, such as strawberries or raspberries

- Two kiwis, plums, or satsumas

- Half a grapefruit or avocado

- 15ml (1 tablespoon) of dried fruit, such as raisins or yellow raisins (sultanas)

- Three dried apricots

- A glass (roughly 100ml / 3½fl.oz) of fruit or vegetable juice

- A small can (roughly 200g/2½oz) of fruit, preferably in natural juice

- A dessert bowl of salad

- Roughly 100g (4oz) of vegetables, such as frozen or mushy peas, boiled carrots, or broccoli

- Roughly 100g (4oz) such as baked beans, kidney beans, peas, or lentils

- The vegetables included in meals like a vegetable curry, lasagne, stir-fry or casserole

Salad days

Salads are a great way to make sure you eat the recommended five fruit and vegetables per day. However choose your dressing carefully. Full-fat mayonnaises, salad creams and dressings will add extra calories. Go for

Take Five

Find it hard to get your five portions of fruit and vegetables every day? Here are some suggestions:

- Drink fruit juice at breakfast
- Add a sliced apple, or banana, or a few strawberries, raspberries or blueberries to your breakfast cereal or oatmeal (porridge)
- Carry a small packet of dried fruit such as raisins, or dried apricots in your bag
- Add salad to sandwiches at lunch time
- Snack on fruit or raw vegetables such as carrots, celery, or peppers. Take some to work. Put them on your desk, so that you're more likely to eat them
- Include at least two vegetables in your evening meal and add fresh fruit to your dessert. It's easy once you make it a habit
- Add grated carrot, zucchini (courgette) or beetroot to your spaghetti bolognese sauce
- Stir-fry chopped vegetables such as peppers, zucchinis (courgettes), mushrooms, onions, carrots or eggplant (aubergine) and add to ready-made tomato or curry sauces
- Add lots of chopped vegetables such as peppers, carrots and onions to home-made curries
- Serve pizza with salad, or homemade coleslaw
- Add a handful of berries or chopped fruit to yogurt, or hot or cold custard, for a quick and healthy pudding
- Add halved strawberries, or slices of melon, mango, or orange, to salads
- If you're too busy to prepare fresh vegetables use frozen ones instead – they're often more nutritious

balsamic vinegar, or swap full-fat dressings for a low-fat version. Or mix ordinary salad cream or mayonnaise with an equal amount of low-fat yogurt for a lower-fat version.

Organic vs non-organic

A growing body of research points to organic fruit and vegetables providing more nutrients than conventionally grown crops. For example, a review by the Food Standards Agency in the UK found that organic vegetables have over 50 percent more beta-carotene than non organic ones. A study at Newcastle University in the UK concluded that organic fruit and vegetables contain 40 percent more antioxidants than non organic. So opt for organic, if you can afford it.

However, non-organic produce is fine so long as you wash or peel it, to reduce any risk from pesticides, before eating.

Beneficial bug boosters

Some foods – mainly fruit and vegetables, contain carbohydrates known as inulins, which feed and stimulate the growth of existing good bacteria in the gut. These are known as prebiotics. They occur naturally in artichokes, onions, garlic, leeks, tomatoes, celery, cucumber, bananas, chickpeas, sunflower seeds and honey. The benefits of eating these foods include better digestive health, increased immunity and improved absorption of calcium.

Get fresh

Ideally fruit and vegetables are best eaten as fresh as possible. Storing them properly helps to retain their nutrients for longer. It's best not to wash fruit and vegetables before putting them in the fridge, as they have a natural coating that helps retain moisture and freshness; washing and scrubbing damages the coating and makes them perish sooner. They also last longer when stored whole. Most vegetables are best stored in perforated plastic or paper bags to help retain moisture – though potatoes are best stored in a cool, dark, dry place.

Carbs – complex and simple!

Carbohydrates are a good source of energy, because they can be converted into glucose more easily than proteins or fats. There are two types of carbohydrate – complex and simple. Complex carbohydrates include cereals, breads, pastas, potatoes and legumes. They provide a slower, steadier release of energy than simple carbohydrates. Refined carbohydrates, such as white bread and white rice, convert into glucose quicker than wholegrains. Carbohydrates should make up about one third of your food intake – though you could need more if you're very active.

The low-down on sugar

Sugars are simple carbohydrates. There are two main types of sugars, monosaccharides and disaccharides. Monosaccharides consist of a single sugar molecule and include glucose, fructose, galactose and fucose. Glucose is found in fruit and vegetables, whilst fructose is found in fruits and honey, and galactose is part of lactose, the sugar found in milk and milk products. Fucose is found in vegetables such as mushrooms, and in kelp.

Disaccharides are sugars composed of two linked up monosaccharide molecules and include sucrose, lactose, and maltose. Sucrose is the refined sugar commonly used in foods and drinks. It's extracted from sugar cane and sugar beet and contains both glucose and fructose. Lactose is found in milk and is made up of glucose and galactose. Maltose is formed when sugars are broken down – for example during beer and whisky production, and is made up of two glucose molecules.

Sugar cravings explained

We crave sweet and starchy foods because the glucose they supply provides vital fuel for both brain and body. When our blood sugar is low, a bar of chocolate or a bag of sweets provides a quick burst of energy. This is because sucrose converts quickly into glucose, which is rapidly absorbed into the bloodstream. When the blood sugar rises too high, too quickly, the body reacts by producing insulin, which lowers it by directing glucose to the body's cells. Our blood sugar then plummets and we crave another sugar 'hit'. Studies even suggest that sugar is addictive and needs to be reduced gradually to prevent withdrawal-type symptoms, such as anxiety.

Sweet enough

For good health and weight management, it's recommended that no more than 10 percent of our energy should come from sugar. There are 20 calories in 5g (1 tsp) of sugar, so for a woman this amounts to 50g (10 tsp) per day. For a man this equates to 62.5g (12½ tsp).

Curb sugar cravings

To beat sugar cravings try sniffing a bottle of vanilla essence. Many find it reduces the urge to eat sweet foods. But eating a diet rich in whole grains, rather than refined foods, is the best way to curb sugar cravings

Sugar – not so sweet!

Over-consumption of sugary foods has been linked to obesity, type 2 diabetes, heart disease and stroke, as well as tooth decay, gum disease and aging skin.

As we've already seen, too much sugar in the diet leads to high blood sugar. This in turn leads to a higher risk of type 2 diabetes.

People who eat a lot of sugar tend to have a low intake of important nutrients, such as Vitamins A and C, folic acid, vitamin B-12, calcium, phosphorous, magnesium and iron. Filling up on sugary foods seems to leave less appetite, or room, for more nutritious foods.

A high consumption of sugar and refined carbohydrates can also result in chromium deficiency. Chromium helps to regulate blood sugar and metabolise fats and carbohydrates. It's found in eggs, meats, seafood, wholegrains, fruit and vegetables.

Natural sweeteners

By contrast, natural sugars found in fruit and vegetables are more complex and are absorbed into the bloodstream more slowly. They're essential for various physiological processes, including immune response and brain function.

For a balanced diet, keep sugary foods and drinks to a minimum. This means avoiding eating too many foods containing refined sugar, such as sugar-coated breakfast cereals, cookies (biscuits), cakes and puddings. Research reveals that manufacturers are adding twice as much sugar to some products than thirty years ago. It's also important to avoid sugary drinks such as cola and lemonade, which can contain up to 35g (7tsp) of sugar per 330ml (½ pt) bottle! Sugar is even added to savory foods, such as soups and sauces.

A diet rich in fruit and vegetables will supply sugars in their natural form, along with other nutrients, whereas sucrose has no nutritional value.

QUICK T!P
SWEETNESS AND LIGHT
If you have a sweet tooth, try to satisfy it with dried fruits, such as raisins, yellow raisins (sultanas), dates, figs, prunes and dried apricots. Fresh fruits, such as ripe bananas, melons and strawberries, are also surprisingly sweet. Once you become accustomed to their natural sweetness, you'll probably find candy, cakes, cookies (biscuits) and desserts too sweet and cloying.

A.K.A. Sugar

When checking food labels for the sugar content of foods, you need to be aware of the other guises it comes under. Any of these terms indicate added sugars. The main ingredients always come first, so if you notice any of these near the top of the list, you know the sugar content is likely to be high.

- Sucrose
- Glucose
- Glucose syrup
- Fructose
- Dextrose
- Golden syrup
- Maple syrup

- Maltose
- Hydrolyzed starch
- Raw sugar
- Corn syrup
- Syrup
- Molasses (Treacle)
- Fruit juice concentrate

- Malt extract
- Invert sugar
- Cane sugar
- Honey
- High fructose corn syrup

Sugar Savers

- Reduce sugar in tea and other beverages gradually, until you can do without
- Use cinnamon or nutmeg to flavor desserts, instead of sugar
- Replace sugar-coated breakfast cereals with wholegrain cereals, or oatmeal (porridge)
- Freeze a banana on a stick, for a sweet but healthy alternative to ice cream
- Choose canned (tinned) fruits in natural juice rather than syrup
- Instead of sweet or stodgy puddings, choose baked apples, summer pudding, or natural yogurt with dried fruit
- Use reduced-sugar jams
- Cut the amount of sugar you use when baking by up to half
- Avoid low fat cookies (biscuits) and bars – they tend to be much higher in sugar, to make them more palatable

Fill up on fiber

High-fiber foods such as whole wheat bread, pasta and rice and fruit and vegetables, fill you up quicker and for longer, tend to be lower in calories and speed up weight loss, because your body burns fat to metabolise fiber.

A diet high in fiber offers numerous health benefits. These include reducing the risk of constipation, piles, diverticular disease, cancers of the bowel and colon, breast cancer in pre-menopausal women, Type 2 diabetes and coronary heart disease.

There are two types of fiber – soluble and insoluble. Both types help to lower blood sugar. Soluble fiber does so by slowing down glucose absorption. Soluble fiber can be partially digested and is found mainly in oats, beans, peas, lentils, and the fleshy part of fruit and vegetables. It's thought to lower cholesterol by absorbing it like a sponge, helping to prevent coronary heart disease. Soluble fiber also acts as a prebiotic, which means it stimulates the growth and activity of beneficial bacteria in the gut. Experts believe this may help relieve inflammatory bowel diseases such as Crohn's disease, ulcerative colitis and clostidrium difficile, a bacterial infection which causes diarrhoea and colitis. It also keeps blood sugar levels stable, by slowing down the rate at which glucose is absorbed into the bloodstream.

Insoluble fiber can't be digested. It helps other food and waste products move through the gut more easily, thus helping to prevent constipation. This fiber is mainly found in wholegrain cereals, brown rice, beans, peas, lentils, oats, and the skins of fruit and vegetables.

It's recommended we eat 18-30g (½–1oz) of fiber daily to enjoy these health benefits.

Fiber and food labels

Current guidelines suggest that a food labelled 'High Fiber' should contain 5g of fiber per serving. A 'good source of fiber' indicates a food providing 2.5 to 4.9g per serving.

Fiber Providers

To help you eat 18-30g of fiber (½–1oz) a day, below are examples of foods which provide approximately 5g (1/8oz) of fiber. In all cases wholegrain versions of cereals, pastas and rice provide the most fiber. The skins of fruit and vegetables are particularly high in insoluble fiber, so eat them whenever possible.

Where appropriate I've compared the amount you'd need to eat of the white, refined version, to gain the same amount of fiber.

- 2 Weetabix – you'd need to eat four 30g (1oz)servings of cornflakes for the same amount of fiber!

- 2 slices wholemeal bread – you'd have to eat 6 slices of white bread

- 3 rye crispbreads

- 150g (5oz) brown rice (uncooked) – you'd need to eat 8 times as much white rice for the same amount of fiber!

- 80g (2½oz) wholewheat pasta (uncooked) – you'd need to eat around three times this amount of white pasta for the equivalent amount of fiber!

- 1 medium baked (jacket) potato (180g/6oz) – including skin. You'd need to eat two and a half times as much mashed potato

- One third of a 415g (14oz) tin of baked beans

- Half a cup of cooked sweetcorn

- 2 medium oranges, pears, apples or bananas

- 45g (3 tablespoons) of frozen peas

Building blocks of life

Protein is necessary for the growth of cells and repair of tissues. All proteins comprise different combinations of 20 compounds known as amino acids. Depending on the amino acids they contain, proteins form enzymes, hormones, muscles, organs and other tissues in the body.

There are two types of amino acids:

- non-essential amino acids – which the body can make

- essential amino acids – which the body can't make and therefore must be obtained from food. There are nine essential amino acids

Protein types

Animal proteins – which contain all the essential amino acids and are found in meat, poultry, fish, eggs and dairy products.

Plant proteins – which contain various amino acids. Sources of plant protein include pulses, cereals, grains, nuts and seeds, soya and Quorn, which contains a vegetable protein obtained from fungus. No one source contains all of the essential amino acids, so if you're vegetarian you need to eat a mix of these foods. For example, beans on toast, or cereal with milk.

QUICK T!P
RED MEAT ALERT
Research has linked a high intake of red, barbequed or processed meats, such as sausages and burgers, to a greater risk of stomach and bowel cancer. A recent study at the Harvard School of Public Health suggested that eating processed meats every day can also increase the risk of heart disease and type 2 diabetes. Plant proteins are low in fat and high in fiber, vitamins, minerals and phytochemicals linked to good health and prevention of illness; so it's best to eat more plant proteins than animal ones.

Protein Providers

To give you an idea of what you'd need to eat to get your recommended daily amounts here's the approximate protein content of some everyday foods:

- One medium egg – 6g (¼oz) of protein

- One skinless chicken breast (130g/4½oz) – 40g (1½oz) of protein

- One small fillet steak (200g/7oz) – 50g (1¾oz) of protein

- One beef burger, or pork sausage – 8g (1/3oz) of protein

- One portion of poached skinless cod fillet (150g/5oz) – 30g (1oz) of protein

- Half a can of tuna – 20g (¾oz) of protein

- One portion of cheese (50g/1¾oz) – 12g (½oz) of protein

- One tablespoon of boiled red lentils (40g/1½oz) – 3g (1/8oz) of protein

- One portion of tofu (125g/ 4½oz) – 15g (½oz) of protein

- One medium slice wholemeal bread – 4g (1/6oz) of protein

- One medium slice white bread – 3g (1/8oz) of protein

- 150ml (1/3pt) glass of milk – 5g (1/5oz) of protein

Protein requirements

It's recommended that we get between 10 and 15 percent of our daily energy intake from protein. This translates into roughly 50 – 75g (2 – 2½ oz) for women and 65 – 95g (2¼ – 3½ oz) for men.

Do dairy

Eat low-fat dairy foods, such as cheese and yogurt, for health benefits linked to their protein and calcium content. Recent research revealed that those who include dairy foods within a weight loss regime lose more weight than those who don't – particularly around the waistline. There are several likely reasons for this. One is that the protein in dairy foods produces a feeling of fullness and stabilizes the blood sugar, reducing sugar cravings and the urge to snack. Another is that milk sugar – lactose, keeps the blood sugar steady, because it converts into glucose more slowly than sucrose.

Also the high calcium content reduces the amount of fat absorbed from foods. Calcium even appears to speed up the rate at which calories are burned.

These benefits appear to halve the risk of developing insulin resistance, a condition where the body doesn't respond properly to insulin. Insulin resistance can result from prolonged high blood sugar levels. It leads to increased cholesterol levels, blood pressure and fat storage, and raises the risk of heart disease, type 2 diabetes and stroke.

Calcium, along with vitamin D, is also necessary for strong bones and the prevention of osteoporosis. Plus it promotes serenity and aids sleep. Studies show it helps prevent PMS and may also ease menopausal symptoms.

The current recommendation is that men and women obtain at least 700mg (1/5oz) of calcium daily from their diet. This equates to roughly 500ml (one pint), of milk, three small tubs of plain, or fruit yogurt, or around 100g (4oz) of hard cheese. Note: Parmesan is rich in calcium and lower in fat than cheddar cheese.

Fat facts

When it comes to eating more healthily and losing weight, most people consider cutting down on the fat content of their diet. Whilst fats are high in energy – 1g (1/16oz) provides 9 calories compared to 4 calories in 1g (1/16oz) of carbohydrate or protein – they are necessary for good health. They're needed for various important functions, including the transportation and absorption of fat-soluble vitamins A, D, E and K, and the cushioning of vital organs. Fats lubricate our skin and gut and help to make food more appetizing too. They also make food more filling, because they slow down glucose absorption – so adding small amounts of beneficial fats can actually help weight management. However, whilst some fats are essential to good health, others are detrimental. Too much of any fat can lead to weight gain. So it's important to ensure you get the correct amounts of the right types of fat.

Healthy fats

The healthiest fats are unsaturated. There are two types of unsaturated fat – polyunsaturated essential fatty acids (omegas 3 and 6) and monounsaturated fat (omega 9).

Essential fatty acids – EFAs – are fats which can't be made by the body and are needed for various functions, including eyesight, healthy skin, hair, and nails, and brain function.

Omega 3s are anti-inflammatory and anti-coagulant and essential for brain development and function. They help protect against cardiovascular disease, arthritis, skin complaints, Huntington's Disease and Multiple Sclerosis. They also appear to help prevent and treat ADHD, dyslexia, depression and other mood disorders and schizophrenia. Health experts in the UK recently recommended that all pupils should be given fish oils to reduce disruptive behavior and improve learning.

Good sources of Omega 3s are:

- Oily fish – pilchards, sardines, salmon, mackerel

- Nuts – especially walnuts, Brazil nuts and almonds

- Seeds – especially sesame

- Oils including soya bean oil, sunflower oil, canola oil, rapeseed oil

- Egg yolks

Omega 6s are also anti-inflammatory and can help prevent and treat a range of conditions; they can ease the symptoms of IBS and promote healthy skin, hair and nails. They promote hormonal balance – relieving and preventing PMS and menopausal symptoms.

Omega 6 fatty acids are found in

- sunflower and corn oils

- olives

- nuts and seeds

- some vegetables and grains

Most people get enough of these in their diet.

Monounsaturated, or **omega 9** fats can lower bad, LDL cholesterol and increase good, HDL cholesterol.

Good sources of omega 9 fats are:

- Olives and olive oil

- Rapeseed oil

- Peanut oil

- Avocados

- Nuts – especially almonds and Brazil nuts

- Seeds – particularly sesame seeds

... and fats to avoid

Saturated fats, otherwise known as hard fats, and mainly found in animal products such as red meat, butter and full-fat dairy foods, such as cheese and milk. Too much saturated fat can raise bad LDL cholesterol levels, which increases the risk of heart disease and atherosclerosis. It may also be linked to some cancers, including breast cancer.

Trans-fats, also known as partially hydrogenated oils, which are mainly found in processed foods. These are formed when liquid vegetable oils are turned into solid fats, through a process called hydrogenation. Trans-fats may be even more detrimental to health than saturated fats. One six-year study showed that monkeys who were fed a diet where 8 percent of the calories came from trans-fats, gained about a fourteenth of their body weight, compared to monkeys fed the same diet – but with mono-unsaturated fats, such as olive oil replacing the trans-fats, who gained less than a fiftieth. The monkeys eating trans-fats also carried about a third more fat on their stomachs, which is a risk factor for heart disease and diabetes.

To reduce saturated and trans fats and increase polyunsaturated and monounsaturated fats in your diet:

- Choose lean meat and trim off visible fat. Remove the skin from roast chicken

- Grill, bake, poach, steam, stew, pressure cook or microwave, rather than fry or roast

- Skim off any fat that rises to the top when cooking stews, or hamburger meat (mince)

- Add more vegetables and less meat to stews and casseroles

- Choose a low-fat accompaniment to a high-fat food, such as meat pie, or pizza, e.g. steamed vegetables, or salad, to achieve a more balanced meal

- Select ready-meals with a lower fat content – check the label. 3 percent of food = low fat. 20 percent = high fat

- Measure oil when cooking, rather than guessing

- When baking cakes replace half the fat with low fat yogurt

- Use a low-fat spread, preferably made with olive oil, rather than butter or full-fat margarine

- Opt for lower-fat dairy foods, such as low-fat yogurts and reduced fat cheeses and reduced fat milk (semi-skimmed) or fat free (skimmed) milk

- Grate cheese, so you use less

- Avoid products with hydrogenated fat, hydrogenated vegetable oil, partially hydrogenated vegetable fat/oil or trans fatty acids listed in the ingredients

- Avoid products with animal/saturated fats, shortening, glycerides, palm oils and milk fats listed in the ingredients

- Choose margarines labelled 'low in trans' or 'virtually trans free'

- Eat oily fish three times a week

- Snack on a handful of nuts or seeds

- Eat hummus – it contains sesame seed paste

- Use olive oil as a salad dressing and in cooking

- Mash potato with olive oil, rather than milk and butter

Fat Checklist

When checking food labels for the fat content of foods, you need to be aware of the guises it comes under. Any of these terms indicate added fats.

- Animal fat

- Butter

- Cocoa butter

- Coconut

- Coconut oil

- Coconut cream

- Egg

- Egg yolk solids

- Lard

- Hydrogenated vegetable oil or fat

- Palm oil

- Palm kernel oil

- Vegetable oil

- Vegetable shortening

- Animal shortening

- Whole milk solids

- Non-milk fat

- Use herbs like basil, mint, or coriander and strong condiments such as mustard, soy sauce and balsamic or white wine vinegar to flavor foods, rather than high-fat sauces and mayonnaises

QUICK T!P
FATS ENOUGH!
Remember, all fats are high in calories, so to ensure a balanced diet and to help maintain a healthy weight it's recommended that no more than a third of our daily energy intake should come from fats. This translates into about 75g (2½oz) for women, of which no more than 20g (¾oz) should be saturated fat and 90g (3½oz) for men, of which no more than 30g (1oz) should be saturated fats.

Swap shop

An easy way to reduce the fat content in your diet is to swap your favorite treats for lower fat, less calorific versions. Here are some ideas to get you started:

- Swap fried or scrambled eggs, for poached or boiled eggs

- Swap pan-fried fries (chips) for oven fries (chips)

- Swap Greek yogurt for low-fat plain yogurt. Low-fat natural set yogurt has a deceptively creamy texture

- Swap chocolate cake for low-fat chocolate mousse

- Swap a bag of potato chips (crisps) for sugar-free popcorn

- Swap ice cream for fruit sorbet

- Swap a croissant for a toasted bagel, with low fat spread

- Swap cheddar cheese for edam

Seasonal swaps

Christmas is a time of indulgence, but it's still possible to eat more healthily and party!

- Swap a sausage roll for a cocktail sausage

- Swap a handful of salted peanuts for a handful of bombay mix

- Swap a handful of potato chips (crisps) for a few olives

- Swap a slice of cheesecake for a portion of pavlova

- Swap a cheese straw for a breadstick

- Swap guacamole for salsa

- Swap cheddar or stilton for brie

Plan for health

Plan your menu for the week ahead before you shop. This helps you achieve a healthier diet because you can decide beforehand which foods you need to buy, rather than grabbing anything that catches your eye. It's much easier to eat a balanced diet if the right ingredients are in the cupboard.

Ready, steady, cook!

Processed foods and ready meals tend to contain more unhealthy fats, sugar and salt. Try preparing meals from basic ingredients for healthier meals. Not only are they more nutritious, they're also far tastier. Try adapting recipes to make them healthier: grill, bake, steam, boil or microwave instead of frying. Use wholemeal flour or part wholemeal flour instead of white. Substitute herbs for salt. Experiment with reducing the amount of sugar in desserts and baking. Some recipes work well with up to half the suggested amount.

No time to cook?

Preparing a healthy meal needn't take a long time. Try roasting vegetables such as peppers, tomatoes, onions and zucchinis (courgettes) in a little olive oil with garlic, chilli and herbs. Add to cooked whole-wheat pasta and stir in a low-fat cream alternative, or a little more olive oil. You could add tuna, or a little Parmesan for added protein. Stir-fries only take minutes to prepare and cook. Broths and casseroles are easy to make – you can do other jobs, once they're on the stovetop (hob), or in the oven. For extra speed, substitute frozen vegetables for fresh. Make your own healthier versions of ready-meals by cooking extra portions of your favorite dishes and freezing them.

Smart snacking

Do you often hit an energy slump mid-morning or afternoon and reach for the cookie (biscuit) tin, a chocolate bar, or bag of potato chips (crisps)? Snacking in itself isn't necessarily a bad thing, depending on the kinds of foods you choose. Junk foods may offer a short-term energy boost, but they're likely to add extra fat, sugar and salt to your diet and few nutrients. If you eat nutritious snacks, they help to maintain your blood sugar levels and provide valuable vitamins, minerals and fiber. Whether at home or at work, always make sure you have a selection of healthy foods to graze on. Fresh fruit, dried fruit, nuts, seeds, carrot or celery sticks, oat cakes, plain digestives, natural yogurt, cottage cheese, crisp breads with peanut butter or hummus, nut or muesli bars and malt loaf, are all excellent snack foods.

Eating out

For more balanced eating out, always opt for small portion sizes. If portions are especially large ask for a child's portion, or order a starter as your main course. Fill up with salad – most restaurants offer salads as starters, or side dishes. Don't be frightened to ask for alternatives to foods on the menu. For example, ask if you can have a baked (jacket) potato, rather than fries (chips), or vegetables and fish, such as tuna or prawns, as a pizza topping.

DINING OUT DO'S & DON'TS

Choose dishes containing the least fat when eating out.

At an Indian restaurant

Many dishes contain a lot of oil or ghee – which is clarified butter – so you need to choose wisely. Avoid deep-fried starters like onion bhajis and samosas. Poppadoms are lower in fat. Lime pickle is high in fat and mango chutney is high in sugar. Opt instead for raita (cucumber dip) or tomato sambai (tomato and onion dip) as an accompaniment.

Forgo creamy curries such as korma, masala or passanda and opt for tandoori, tikka, or madras dishes, with boiled rice and chapatti, or tandoori roti, rather than pilau rice and naan, which are quite high in fat. Other lower-fat dishes include aloo gobi, vegetable curry and aloo saag. Dahl or dhansak are healthy choices, as they contain fiber-rich lentils.

At an Italian restaurant

Eat dishes with tomato, rather than cream-based sauces, and choose lower-fat pizza toppings such as vegetables, prawns or ham. Instead of garlic bread, try bruschetta – a ciabatta bread with a tomato and herb topping.

In a Chinese restaurant

Avoid foods in batter, as they're high in fat. Go for lower-fat options, such as stir-fries with boiled rice or noodles, chicken chop suey or Szechuan dishes.

In a Thai restaurant

Avoid battered foods. Choose stir-fried or steamed dishes with jasmine rice, rather than egg-fried. Thai green and red curries contain coconut milk, making them high in fat, so eat them in moderation.

At a Japanese restaurant

Choose sushi and stir-fries. Again avoid battered dishes such as tempura. Japanese banquets tend to consist of small portions of various foods including salads, fish, chicken and miso soups and on the whole provide fairly healthy and balanced cuisine.

At a Mexican restaurant

Select salsa with fajitas, rather than sour cream. Salsa is low in fat and contains phytonutrients.

Better burgers and kebabs

At a burger bar choose grilled rather than fried and opt for those made from lean meat or fish. Say 'no' to cheese or mayonnaise and ask for a wholemeal bun and extra salad. If you enjoy a kebab go for chicken, rather than lamb, which is much fattier. Add salad and chilli sauce, rather than garlic mayonnaise, for a lower-fat and more balanced meal.

At the fish and chip shop

To make fish and fries (chips) a healthier option, don't eat all of the batter, as it soaks up a lot of fat, or go for fish in breadcrumbs, which absorbs less fat. Try a smaller portion of fries (chips) or share them. Another tip is to blot the fat from your meal using paper towel (kitchen roll). But be aware that fried fish and fries are high in fat and are best eaten only occasionally if you're serious about being healthy. Or you could forgo the fish shop altogether and opt for the lower-fat alternative of oven baked frozen fries (chips) and oven baked fish in bread crumbs. Serve with peas, green beans, or broad beans for a more nutritious meal. Finally, avoid adding salt if you can. But go ahead with the traditional sprinkling of vinegar, because it helps you absorb certain minerals and keeps your blood sugar steady.

Healthier sandwiches

Choose brown, granary or wholemeal bread for extra fiber. Select low fat fillings such as lean meat, tuna, prawns, hard boiled egg or cheese such as Edam, Emmental, Gruyere, or low fat cream cheese. For extra vitamins go for added salad. If the sandwich is made to order, opt for no, or only a little butter, margarine, or mayonnaise, or go for lower-fat versions. Avoid full-fat mayonnaise, choose low-fat salad dressings, salsa, or mustard instead.

When buying pre-packed sandwiches, check the label for the fat content. Choose sandwiches with 3 percent fat and 1 percent saturated fat or less, if possible.

Saline solution

A high intake of salt is linked with high blood pressure and the risk of coronary heart disease, stroke, stomach cancer, osteoporosis, kidney problems and even stomach ulcers. Current guidelines urge us to eat no more than 6g (¼oz) of salt daily, but this can be hard to achieve if you eat a lot of processed and pre-packaged foods. For example, pre-packed sandwiches can contain between 2.5g (1/16oz) and 4g (1/6oz) of salt and a tin of a well-known brand's 'healthy' lentil and bacon soup contains 4g (1/6oz). A 400g (140z) tin of regular baked beans contains 5g (1/8oz) of salt.

Doctors claim that many lives could be saved each year if we all stuck to the recommended limit. The best way to reduce salt in your diet is to eat meals prepared and cooked at home, using little or no salt. Try flavoring your cooking with herbs. Use lime, garlic, ginger and chillis in stir-fries. Squeeze lemon juice on fish and seafood. Use black pepper on pasta and eggs. Olives and pickled capers are also good for adding flavor to pastas, pizzas and salads.

When cooking from scratch isn't possible, check food labels for salt content. But beware, many food manufacturers give the sodium content, which has to be multiplied by 2.5 to calculate the salt content. Plus, often the sodium or salt content per 100g is provided, which again necessitates arithmetic to work out the total amount in a product.

Products listing any of the following among their ingredients are likely to be high in salt:

- Monosodium glutamate
- Disodium phosphate
- Brine
- Garlic salt
- Onion salt
- Sodium benzoate
- Sodium alginate
- Sodium hydroxide
- Sodium caseinate
- Sodium hydroxide
- Sodium nitrate
- Sodium pectinate
- Sodium propianate
- Sodium sulphite
- Soy sauce
- Baking powder
- Baking soda

Food labels – a quick & easy guide

Ingredients, including additives, have to be listed in descending order of weight, so it's easy to spot the main ones.

Some food manufacturers use traffic light colors on the front of food products to help you identify if the food has low, medium or high levels of fat sugar and salt. Green indicates low, amber medium and red high. So the more green lights on a product, the healthier it is, in terms of fat, sugar and salt levels.

Many food companies display the calories and grams of sugars, fats and salt in a serving of food, and how this measures up as a percentage of your Guideline Daily Amounts/ Daily Values. These are based on the energy and nutrient requirements of an average adult.

A downside is that the figures given are often for servings much smaller than those people actually eat. Also people's dietary needs vary according to their age, sex and levels of activity. However, they do help you to make sensible food choices. As a general guide 5 percent or less of your Guideline Daily Amounts/Daily Values is low, whilst 20 percent or more is high.

Hidden extras

Many processed foods are high in added sugar, fat or salt – all of which can lead to weight gain and health problems. Low-fat products often contain excessive amounts of added sugar. For example, a yogurt containing only 2.7g of fat per 100g is labelled low-fat, suggesting it's a healthy food choice. Yet it contains 15.7g of sugar per 100g – 19.6 g per pot, which equals nearly 4 teaspoons.

Breakfast cereals are viewed as a healthy start to the day, yet they're often high in sugar, salt and fat. For instance, a well-known supermarket's own-brand crunchy oat cereal contains 20.3g of fat per 100g. Some savory sauces and pizzas contain added sugar.

So choose foods with as few additives as possible. For example natural unsweetened yogurt – you can add some dried fruit to sweeten it, if necessary. Plain oatmeal (porridge), or shredded wheat, have no hidden extras, making them a healthier choice.

Don't be misled!

Food labels can be very misleading. Here's a brief guide to commonly used terms and what they actually mean.

Strawberry flavor doesn't mean a product contains strawberries, however strawberry flavored does. Also, if there's a picture of strawberries on the wrapper, the item must contain them. But check the label, as the strawberry content could be very low.

Words such as original, healthy, authentic, wholesome, nutritious, selected and real, mean nothing at all, as there is no legal definition for them.

Light or 'lite' doesn't mean a product is low in fat. It usually means the product is lower in fat than the standard version, but it could still contain more fat than the standard version from another brand.

Reduced fat doesn't mean low fat. The term can be used to describe a food that contains 25 percent less fat than the standard version. The food could still be high in fat. The same applies to reduced sugar, sodium and energy! Often a reduced fat product has added sugar to make it more palatable, so the calories it contains remain the same as the standard version.

Fat-free doesn't equal low in fat. For example if a product states it's 92 percent fat free, that means it contains 8 percent fat, which makes it a medium-fat food.

Low cholesterol means 20mg or less per serving but the product could still be high in fat.

No added sugar means no added sucrose, but other types of sugar, such as glucose or fructose could have been used instead.

Natural, or made from natural, simply means that the manufacturer made the product using ingredients from a natural source. After processing, these ingredients may bear little resemblance to their original state!

Free from artificial preservatives may mean a product contains other additives that extend shelf life, such as salt or sugar.

Farm fresh or country fresh eggs may bear an image of a hen scratching around a farmyard, but in all likelihood they'll have been produced by battery hens. Free-range eggs must come from hens with access to the outdoors. Barn eggs come from hens that live indoors, but have freedom of movement and access to perches and nests. Organic eggs are guaranteed to have been laid by uncaged hens, allowed to roam on organic pasture.

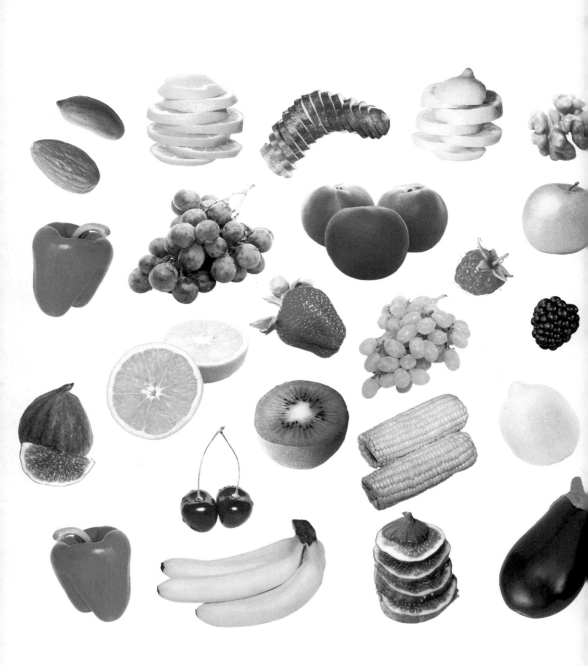

Superfoods

" Let your medicine be your food and your food be your medicine. "

Hippocrates

Chapter 4
Superfoods

Superfoods deliver a high concentration of health-boosting nutrients. However, remember the key to a healthy diet is to eat a variety of foods, as no one food can provide all of the nutrients your body needs. If your current diet is based on processed foods, you'll reap huge health benefits by gradually introducing some of these 'super foods'. None are expensive or exotic – they are ordinary, everyday foods that can be bought at your local supermarket.

A handful of almonds

Eating a handful of almonds daily reduces CHD, cancer and diabetes risk factors and has an anti-aging effect. Almonds contain 20 flavonoids, vitamin E and monounsaturated fat, as well as protein, fiber and minerals. Flavonoids are plant pigments that have an antioxidant effect on the body, protecting cells from damage and preventing clogged arteries. Almonds also appear to boost weight loss. It seems that the protein, fat and fiber keep you full longer and not all of the calories they contain are absorbed, because of their tough cell walls. Finally, almonds are good for your bones, as they are rich in calcium.

An apple a day …

An apple a day does indeed keep the physician away. Evidence suggests that apples are an all-round health booster. They appear to act as 'magic bullets' against various cancers, as well as reducing blood cholesterol and providing various vitamins and minerals. Apples contain the flavonoid quercetin, an antioxidant that boosts the immune system, helping to reduce the risk of illnesses ranging from the common cold, to breast, colon and prostrate cancers and heart disease. The skins contain phytonutrients (plant nutrients) thought to reduce the growth of colon cancer cells by 43 percent. Other flavonoids in apples appear to reduce the risk of lung and bladder cancers.

Research shows that eating five or more apples a week can improve lung function and reduce the risk of asthma in adults. Children whose mothers eat apples during pregnancy are less likely to develop asthma. This may be down to the antioxidants counteracting the effects of pollution and easing inflammation.

Apples also contain pectin, a soluble fiber that mops up cholesterol. Crunching into an apple cleans between your teeth and massages your gums, promoting dental health. Finally, fresh apples are a decent source of vitamin C and, because of their low Glycemic Index, help you to maintain a healthy weight.

Go bananas

Bananas not only provide energy, they also protect against strokes, heart disease, stomach ulcers and anemia, as well as reducing stress and depression. Bananas are high in potassium which helps maintain sodium levels in the body and prevent high blood pressure. They also contain tryptophan and vitamin B6, which are used by the body to make mood-enhancing serotonin.

Beet it!

Beetroot acts as a blood purifier, boosts immunity and has anti-cancer properties. It's a good source of folic acid, which may protect against Alzheimer's, dementia and high blood pressure and helps maintain a good supply of red blood cells. Folic acid is essential during early pregnancy to prevent spinal cord defects, such as spina bifida. Liver is the best source, but isn't recommended during pregnancy, due to it containing high levels of vitamin A, which can harm the baby. A 100g (4oz) serving of beetroot contains 75 percent of the recommended daily intake of folic acid. Beetroot also contains iron – again needed for healthy blood and silica – essential for healthy tendons, ligaments, bones, fingernails, skin and hair. It's low in calories, contains soluble fiber and has a 'medium' Glycemic Index, so it helps to keep blood sugar levels stable.

It's also thought to lower homocysteine levels in the blood. Homocysteine is an amino acid produced by the body when it breaks down methionine, another amino acid. A high level in the blood indicates a high risk of developing diseases such cardiovascular disease, dementia, osteoporosis and problems in pregnancy. Eating foods rich in folic acid and vitamins B6 & 12 lowers homocysteine to a safer level. Other foods rich in folic acid include green leafy vegetables, citrus fruits, pulses and wholegrain cereals.

Finally, drinking beetroot juice daily has been shown to improve stamina, enabling people to exercise for longer. It's thought that beetroot juice's energy boosting properties are due to its high nitrate levels, which improve the supply of oxygen to the muscles.

Berry good for you!

Berries such as blueberries, blackberries, blackcurrants, cranberries, raspberries and strawberries, contain a wealth of health-promoting vitamins, minerals and phytochemicals. A serving of ten strawberries provides the recommended daily allowance of folic acid.

Berries are generally a good source of vitamins C and E and anthocyanins, powerful antioxidants, which are anti-aging, anti-cardiovascular disease, anti-cancer and antibacterial. Anthocyanins are plant pigments – the darker the fruit, the more it contains, so fruits such as blackcurrants, blueberries and blackberries are rich sources. Cranberries also contain beneficial amounts.

A recent study in New Zealand claimed that an antioxidant found in blackcurrants called epigallocatechin can help asthma sufferers by easing breathing and reducing lung inflammation.

Research suggests that the vitamins and anthocyanins in berries can prevent age-related brain deterioration and can even improve short-term memory and restore coordination in those already affected. They may also keep eyes healthy, reducing eyestrain, improving night vision and helping to prevent age-related macular degeneration (AMD) – a common cause of blindness in the over 50s.

Anthocyanins are also effective against E.coli – a common cause of stomach upsets, diarrhea and cystitis. Some berries, such as blueberries and cranberries, also contain a substance which discourages this bacteria from sticking to the mucous membranes of the bladder and uretha, again helping to prevent urinary tract infections. H.pylori, a cause of stomach ulcers, is also prevented from adhering to the stomach lining. Anthocyanins may also prevent the excessive growth of fungi in the body, such as Candida albicans, which often causes vaginal infections and has been linked with IBS. They seem to inhibit the growth of the bacteria which cause gum disease, helping to promote better oral health.

Another antioxidant found in berries, ellagic acid, is believed to prevent cancers, by restricting cancer cell growth. Raspberries contain the highest amounts.

Berries are also rich in the soluble fiber pectin, which lowers cholesterol. Their seeds are beneficial too – providing essential fatty acids. Studies suggest that blackcurrants are the most nutritious berries, followed by blueberries, raspberries and strawberries.

Brain-boosting Brazils

Like other nuts, Brazil nuts are packed with essential vitamins and minerals. They are an excellent source of selenium, which is believed to protect against Alzheimer's, depression and cancer. Recent research suggested that eating a few Brazil nuts daily can help reduce the risk of various cancers, including cancer of the liver, lungs, stomach and prostrate.

They're rich in Omega-3 and Omega-6 fatty acids and oleic acid and contain vitamin E, which is antioxidant and anti-aging. They also contain linoleic acid, important for the skin and hormone balance.

QUICK T!P
CARROTS ARE TOPS!
Carrots are a good source of the antioxidant beta-carotene. To gain the most benefit, roast carrots in a healthy fat, such as olive oil. Roasting softens the cell walls, making the beta-carotene more digestible. Adding fat helps the body to absorb it. Alternatively, boil or steam carrots whole, as this helps to retain nutrients and flavor. Studies suggest that a natural pesticide in carrots, called falcarinol, may lower the risk of developing cancer. They also contain soluble fiber.

Red hot chilli peppers

High in vitamin A and the antioxidant beta-carotene, chilli peppers also contain capsaicin, which gives them their heat, and may stop the spread of prostrate and pancreatic cancer cells. Capsaicin also prevents and treats stomach ulcers, because it reduces acid and increases alkali, as well as improving blood circulation in the stomach. Excessive amounts of hot chillies has been linked to stomach cancer, so don't overdo them.

Chilli peppers seem to keep blood insulin levels steady, so may reduce the risk of type 2 diabetes.

Consuming dishes containing chilli regularly appears to burn fat cells and raise the metabolism. Chillis are also anti-inflammatory, bringing relief to arthritis sufferers, and may help prevent arteriosclerosis. They stimulate the release of 'feel good' brain chemicals, endorphins, which also have a pain-relieving effect.

QUICK T!P

INDULGE IN A LITTLE DARK CHOCOLATE

Indulging in a little dark chocolate could boost your health and help you lose weight! Studies show that good quality dark chocolate (made with 70 percent or more cocoa) contains flavonols which are antioxidants that have a clot-busting and blood-pressure lowering effect. They also appear to boost blood flow to the brain, thus improving brain function and counteracting fatigue. Dark chocolate also increases mood and sleep-enhancing serotonin in the brain, which helps to curb the appetite. It has a low Glycemic Index too, so it keeps you feeling full for longer. Milk chocolate contains fewer flavonols and more fat and sugar. For maximum health benefits eat about one to two ounces daily, as even dark chocolate can be high in fat and sugar!

Get cracking!

Eggs are nutritional powerhouses supplying vitamins A, D and E, as well as the minerals calcium, iodine, iron, phosphorous, selenium and zinc. They are rich in B vitamins, especially B2, B12, folate, biotin, pantothenic acid and choline. B vitamins are needed for various functions in the body, including the release of energy from food, a healthy nervous system and blood formation. An excellent source of protein, eggs provide nine essential amino acids. They also contain the antioxidants lutein and zeaxanthin, which are thought to protect against two causes of sight loss – cataracts and age-related macular degeneration (AMD). Eggs used to have a bad press because of their cholesterol content, but it's now generally agreed that saturated fats have more influence on cholesterol levels than cholesterol in food; eggs are low in saturated fat. They're also low in salt. The healthiest way to eat them is either boiled or poached.

Grape expectations

Eating red, purple, or black grapes could prevent a host of illnesses and even help you sleep better! They contain resveratrol, an antioxidant believed to improve blood flow to the brain, protect against thrombosis (clots) and arteriosclerosis (hardening of the arteries), balance hormones and prevent breast and prostrate cancers and osteoporosis . Other antioxidants in grapes are believed to reduce cholesterol levels, prevent Alzheimer's, gum disease, colds and allergies and benefit arthritis. Grapes are thought to contain melatonin, a hormone which helps regulate the sleep cycle. They also contain the antioxidant procyanidin, which is also thought to prevent thrombosis and arteriosclerosis, as well cut the risk of mouth and lung cancers and reduce skin inflammation associated with eczema. Eat seeded grapes – the darker the better – as these contain the most procyanidin.

Eat your greens

Green vegetables such as broccoli, Brussels sprouts, cauliflower and cabbage contain antioxidant vitamins A and C and vitamin B complex, including folic acid. Folic acid is especially important in early pregnancy when it helps prevent neural tube defects, such as spina bifida.

Dark green vegetables are also rich in vitamin K, which helps to keep bones strong by regulating calcium levels and promoting blood clotting. Eat dark green vegetables in moderation if you take warfarin to prevent blood clotting, as too much Vitamin K could affect the drug's effectiveness. Broccoli and purple sprouting broccoli are rich in vitamin C. One portion contains the recommended daily amount. Broccoli also contains the natural phytoestrogen (plant estrogen) lignan, believed to help protect against breast cancer and relieve menopausal symptoms.

Leafy green vegetables are a good source of iron. Iron comes in two different forms, haem, from meat, and non-haem, from plants. Non-haem is harder for the body to absorb. Vitamin C aids absorption, making leafy green vegetables particularly good for vegetarians and vegans. Broccoli, kale and spinach are also rich in the antioxidants beta-carotene and lutein. Beta-carotene protects against various cancers and UV light. Lutein reduces the risk of age-related macular degeneration (AMD), which can lead to blindness. It also protects the eyes from UV damage and cataracts. Eating these vegetables with a small amount of fat, such as olive oil, helps your body to absorb the lutein.

Green vegetables are thought to have anti-cancer properties, due to their glucosinolate content. Glucosinolates are compounds containing glucose and sulfur. They give vegetables like Brussels sprouts their bitter taste. How we store and cook our greens can have a marked effect on the glucosinolate content.

QUICK T!P
FRESH BEATS FROZEN
Freezing and thawing green vegetables cuts the glucosinolate content by a third. Storing fresh vegetables in the fridge or at room temperature for a week has little effect.

Slice, don't shred

Finely shredding green vegetables also destroys glucosinolates. So slice or tear instead.

Steam or stir-fry

Boiling green vegetables dramatically lowers the glucosinolate, vitamin C and folic acid content. Microwaving in a little water is better, but steaming and stir-frying preserve the most nutrients.

Let's have lettuce

Boost your intake of vitamins and minerals by adding a couple of handfuls of lettuce leaves to your meals. The darker the leaves, the more nutrients they contain; romaine lettuce, an ingredient of Caesar salad, is rich in cancer fighting beta – carotene. It's also a good source of vitamin C and lutein, both of which protect against age-related macular degeneration (AMD). The dark red hues of Lollo Rosso are down to its antioxidant content, which is100 times higher than that of other salad leaves, according to researchers at Glasgow University. One of the antioxidants it contains, quercetin, is thought to protect against allergies, including hay fever and asthma. Lambs lettuce provides beta-carotene, vitamin C and folate. Folate helps to protect against neural tube defects, such as spina bifida, when eaten during pregnancy.

Have hazel nuts

Just fifteen hazel nuts provide the recommended daily intake of vitamin E for women. Vitamin E protects the body from the effects of pollution, stress and the sun. They may also help prevent cataracts and Alzheimer's.

A taste of honey

If you have a sweet tooth, try replacing sugar with honey, which is a healthier alternative, because it contains amino acids, vitamins, minerals and antioxidants. Honey contains a mixture of fructose, glucose, maltose, sucrose and other sugars, which are formed from nectar by an enzyme produced by bees. A natural source of sugars, it's an instant energy-booster, but has a gentler and longer-lasting effect on blood sugar levels than sugar.

It also provides trace amounts of B vitamins, and various minerals, including calcium, iron, zinc, potassium and chromium. The presence of selenium, vitamin C, enzymes and flavonoids, gives honey its antioxidant properties. Researchers recently concluded that honey has a mild cholesterol-lowering effect.

If you suffer from hayfever, try eating one teaspoon of honey produced within a five mile radius of where you live, every day. There is anecdotal evidence that the pollen in the honey will boost your immunity to the allergens that cause your hayfever. However remember that honey is still a form of sugar, so try not to eat more than two or three teaspoons daily.

Mushroom magic

Mushrooms seem to lower estrogen levels, which may help reduce the risk of breast cancer. They may cut the risk of prostrate cancer by inhibiting enzymes linked with its development. They're rich in antioxidants and the immunity-boosting trace-mineral selenium. They contain insoluble fiber and a natural statin called lovastatin, both of which lower cholesterol, helping to reduce the risk of CHD. They're also rich in blood-pressure-lowering potassium. Finally, mushrooms are a good source of B vitamins, including folic acid.

Have you had your oats?

Oats contain a soluble fiber called beta glucan, which lowers blood cholesterol, cutting the risk of heart disease. Rich in insoluble fiber they have a low Glycemic Index, making oatmeal (porridge) a great breakfast to help manage your weight. Plus they're a good source of chromium, which balances blood sugar, as well as iron, zinc, manganese,vitamin E, thiamin and folate.

Not just cool for cats!

Oily fish such as salmon, sardines, herrings, mackerel, trout and tuna are not just high in protein, they also contain up to eight times as much health-boosting omega-3 and omega-6 fatty acids as lean fish, such as cod, haddock, monkfish and sole.

Sprats contain the most, followed by salmon, sardines, mackerel and herring. Fresh tuna and trout are also decent sources. They're also a good source of vitamin E and the mineral selenium. Canned oily fish with edible bones, such as salmon and sardines, are a good source of calcium too.

Love olive oil

Olive oil features heavily in the Mediterranean diet, which is believed to reduce the risk of heart disease, stroke, cancer and arthritis. It's rich in monounsaturated fats, which lower blood cholesterol and a good source of Vitamin E, which thins the blood, boosts immunity and acts as an antioxidant. Evidence that olive oil reduces the risk of breast, skin and colon cancer is attributed to other components, such as oleic acid and phenols. It is also thought to reduce inflammation, which benefits arthritis sufferers, reducing joint pain and stiffness and improving grip strength. Its anti-inflammatory properties have been attributed to a chemical found in olive oil called oleocanthal. Eating vegetables cooked in olive oil is thought to reduce the risk of developing rheumatoid arthritis. Its sweet, slightly spicy flavor makes it a great dip for fresh crusty brown bread, or a tasty salad dressing.

Know your onions

Like apples, onions contain quercetin, but absorption from onions is three times greater. Like garlic, onions contain good levels of allicin. They're also a good source of chromium, which helps stabilise blood sugar, maintain hormonal balance and prevent PMS. Finally, they're natural pre-biotics, which promote the growth of 'good' bacteria in the gut.

Opt for oranges

Oranges are high in vitamin C and the phytonutrient hesperitin, which appears to discourage breast cancer cell growth. Eating oranges and other citrus fruits seems to reduce the risk of both stomach and skin cancers.

Peanut power

Peanuts contain soluble and insoluble fiber, which are good for the digestion and lowering cholesterol. They're high in protein and a good source of polyunsaturated and monounsaturated fats. More than 75 percent of the total fat content is unsaturated. They contain the amino acid arginine, resveratrol (also found in red wine), plant sterols and other phytochemicals, which are thought to have cardio-protective and cancer-preventing properties. They're cholesterol free and contain minerals such as zinc, magnesium, copper and selenium, plus vitamin Bs, folate and vitamin E. Eating peanut butter seems to aid weight loss – probably because of its low Glycemic Index. For the healthiest option, choose peanut butter without hydrogenated fat.

QUICK T!P
THE HUMBLE POTATO
Potatoes are cheap, filling, nutritious and low in fat, if you bake or boil them and don't add too much butter or margarine. They contain carbohydrate, protein and fiber. They're also a good source of B vitamins, including B6 and folic acid and provide vitamin C. High in potassium, they can help lower blood pressure.

Take your pulse

Pulses, also known as legumes, include beans, peas and lentils. They have anti-cancer properties – not only due to their fiber content, but also because they contain compounds that inhibit tumor growth. A good source of protein, slow-release carbohydrate, soluble and insoluble fiber, vitamins and minerals, pulses are a valuable addition to anyone's diet. They count as one portion of vegetables.

Haricot beans, most often eaten as baked beans, are the most popular. Baked beans are an excellent source of iron and folic acid and also provide calcium. The ketchup (tomato sauce) provides lycopene. For the healthiest option, go for low salt and sugar versions.

Red kidney beans, an ingredient of the popular mexican dish, chilli con carne, contain a substance which can upset the stomach. Either boil for fifteen minutes and then drain before use, or for ease, use the canned (tinned) versions.

Soya beans supply all of the essential amino acids, making them the only pulse to provide first class plant protein. They're also the best food source of isoflavones, plant hormones which reduce menopausal symptoms and the risk of breast cancer in women. Soya also reduces the risk of prostrate and colon cancers and lowers cholesterol.

Lentils are especially high in fiber – a 200g (7oz) portion contains around 16g – almost the recommended daily amount.

Peas contain lutein, an antioxidant believed to protect eye health.

Remember rhubarb

A recent study in the UK concluded that baked rhubarb can help to prevent the growth of cancer cells. Baking rhubarb for 20 minutes increases the levels of cancer-preventing antioxidants called polyphenols. It is a good source of vitamin K and minerals – especially calcium and contains both soluble and insoluble fiber.

Ex-seedingly good

Seeds, including sunflower, sesame and pumpkin, make a great snack. They're rich in protein and Essential Fatty Acids, as well as vitamins B and E and minerals – especially magnesium. Their high EFA content means they promote hormonal balance, helping to prevent PMS.

Sweet potato sustenance

Sweet potatoes are even more nutritious than white potatoes and have a lower Glycemic Index, so they keep you full for longer. They contain three times as much vitamin C as a regular potato and nearly twice as much beta-carotene as carrots. Unlike white potatoes sweet potatoes count towards your 'five a day'.

Select sweet peppers

Peppers are rich in fiber and high in vitamin C, beta-carotene and potassium. They also contain the sight-protecting plant pigments lutein and zeaxanthin. Researchers at the University of Wisconsin suggested recently that these substances are absorbed by the eyes, where they protect against the harmful effects of UV radiation. The vitamin C they contain is thought to help prevent cataracts. Red peppers, which are ripened green peppers, contain the most nutrients, including decent amounts of lycopene, an antioxidant that gives them their red color. Eat peppers raw in salads or lightly stir-fried, to get the maximum amount of vitamin C. Cooking them in oil enables your body to absorb more beta-carotene and lycopene.

Tomato sauce

Having tomato-based sauces on pasta and other dishes may help to protect against heart disease, cancer, skin damage from the sun, and maintain eye health. Tomatoes are the richest source of lycopene, which is thought to prevent prostrate and other cancers by neutralizing free radicals (substances produced by the body when dealing with exposure to pollutants, such as cigarette smoke, overexposure to sunlight and illness) believed to cause cell damage. Lycopene may also help to keep eyes healthy and functioning well. Cooking tomatoes releases lycopene from the tomato cell walls, making it easier for the body to absorb. Lycopene dissolves in fat, so eating cooked tomatoes in the form of purees or sauce, with a source of fat such as cheese or olive oil, helps with absorption. So pizza, preferably served with a mixed salad, can be a healthy meal.

Wonderful walnuts

Walnuts appear to undo some of the harmful effects of eating saturated fats.

As well as being a good source of omega 3s, walnuts contain arginine, an amino acid, and antioxidants. Research shows they can reduce hardening of the arteries – arteriosclerosis, caused by saturated fats. Arteriosclerosis reduces blood flow through the arteries over time. It's thought the arginine is used by the body to make nitric oxide, which is needed to maintain the flexibility and elasticity of the arteries. This means the arteries can expand when needed, for increased blood flow. Walnuts are rich in monounsaturated fats, which means they lower cholesterol too. But don't assume that eating walnuts can make up for a diet high in saturated fats! Aim at reducing saturated fats as well. To gain the most benefit eat them raw.

Say 'yes' to yogurt

Eating live bio-yogurt provides 'good' bacteria to boost your immune system and may even help you to control your weight. Known as probiotics, these bacteria also have anti-inflammatory properties, which help combat the symptoms of irritable bowel syndrome (IBS) and inflammatory bowel disease. They appear to treat diarrhea in children, as well as relieving the symptoms of lactose intolerance and possibly reducing the risk of colo-rectal cancer. They also help to beat bad breath. Recent research suggests that probiotics cut levels of 'bad bacteria' in the gut, which are thought to increase both our absorption of the calories in our food and their storage as fat. Choose yogurts that contain the bacteria strains bifidobacteria, lactobacilli or streptococcus thermophilus, as these are thought to be the most beneficial.

Make way for watercress

Watercress is rich in the antioxidants, beta-carotene, lutein and zeaxanthin, and vitamins B1, B6 C, E and K, as well as iron, magnesium and zinc. A daily serving may cut your risk of getting cancer by reducing damage to white blood cells and boosting their ability to resist damage by free radicals. It's also thought to be good for thyroid function because it contains decent amounts of iodine.

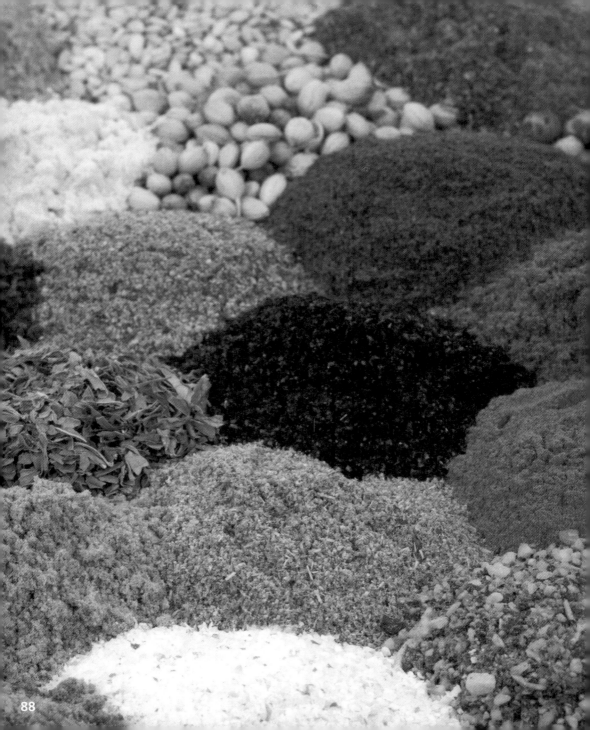

Spice of Life

66 Once you have a spice in your home, you have it forever. Women never throw out spices. **99**

Emma Lombeck

Chapter 5
Spice of Life

Spices are usually extracted from the bark, stem and seeds of plants. They not only add flavor to your food, but also offer a variety of health benefits when consumed regularly. Even a pinch is enough to make a difference, because of the potent chemicals spices contain, such as isothiocyanates, natural compounds which seem to inhibit cancers.

Amazing anise seed

Anise seed is the liquorice-flavored seed of the anise plant, a member of the carrot family. It is used in Ayurvedic medicine as a carminative – which means it can both prevent the formation of wind (gas) and ease the passing of it. Herbalists have traditionally used it to ease griping pains and help digestion. It is thought to regulate the digestive system, making it useful for all types of irritable bowel syndrome (IBS). It also has soothing, sedative properties. Its expectorant action makes it helpful for bronchitis. The active constituent is trans-anethole, which is responsible for the distinctive flavor and smell of aniseed. The seeds can be chewed, or used to make a tea. Lightly crush the seeds first and then pour boiling water over them. Leave to brew for about five minutes. Strain and drink.

A pinch of black pepper

Black pepper stimulates the taste buds, which promote the secretion of hydrochloric acid in the stomach, improving digestion. It's reported to boost circulation and is antibacterial. It helps prevent water retention by promoting sweating and having a diuretic effect. It may help your body break down fats.

Clot buster

Researchers in India recently reported that cardamom has anti-blood-clotting properties, which means it could reduce the risk of heart attack and stroke. Chewing cardamom seeds also eases flatulence, colic and indigestion.

Cayenne soother

Cayenne is a hot, fiery spice made from ground chilli pods and seeds. It offers many of the benefits of chillis, such as relieving pain, boosting the circulation and reducing blood clotting. Despite its fieriness, like chillis, it's reputed to soothe stomach ulcers and ease indigestion.

A sprinkle of cinnamon

Sprinkling cinnamon on food and drinks can help prevent serious disease, as well as treat minor complaints. One teaspoon of ground cinnamon is thought to provide the same amount of antioxidants as 80g of blueberries. It stimulates the circulation, helping to reduce blood stickiness, which can cause clots, strokes and heart attacks. It's also good for the digestion, relieving nausea, flatulence and diarrhea. The smell of cinnamon is thought to stimulate brain activity and have an aphrodisiac effect.

A compound in this spice helps your body convert glucose into energy more easily, which helps to stabilise blood sugar levels. Studies suggest it may help prevent and treat type 2 diabetes. It's also thought to reduce cholesterol and triglyceride levels. Cinnamon may boost the metabolism and ease joint stiffness and pain too.

It tastes great sprinkled on a cappuccino or latte. Try it sprinkled on toast, oatmeal (porridge), or sweet potato. It adds flavor to apple crumble and baked apples.

Calming cloves

Cloves contain various nutrients including Vitamin C, calcium and omega 3 oils. They're thought to soothe the stomach and ease nausea and vomiting. They also contain eugenol, which has an anesthetic effect and is antiseptic and anti-inflammatory, relieving toothache and inflammatory conditions, such as arthritis. They're traditionally used to treat respiratory conditions such as bronchitis and asthma. Cloves add flavor to vegetable and fruit dishes, as well as to soups, curries and mulled wine.

Make room for cumin

Cumin seeds are a good source of iron and manganese. They promote digestion by stimulating the release of pancreatic enzymes and relieve flatulence, colic and diarrhea. They're also thought to prevent muscle cramps. In Ayurvedic medicine they are used to relieve morning sickness and stimulate milk production. Cumin also contains thymoquinone, an antioxidant with anti-inflammatory properties that may help to ease arthritis pain.

Seek fenugreek

Fenugreek seeds have been shown to help weight loss. It's thought the fiber they contain keeps you feeling full for longer and stabilizes blood sugar levels, which also benefits people with both type 1 and 2 diabetes.

They also settle indigestion and soothe allergies. They contain saponins, natural detergents believed to lower cholesterol and triglyceride levels in the blood. Historically they've been used to treat bronchitis, arthritis, wounds and absesses. In Chinese medicine they're used to treat kidney problems.

Fenugreek can stimulate the uterus, so it's not advised during pregnancy, in case of miscarriage. Evidence suggests it may stop, or slow the growth of breast cancer.

Gain from garlic

Garlic contains sulfur compounds called diallyl sulfides and allicin, which are believed to fight viral and bacterial infections, boost immunity, prevent thrombosis, lower cholesterol and the risk of stomach and bowel cancers and protect against heart attacks and strokes. Leave crushed or chopped garlic for about ten minutes to 'mature' before cooking, to help prevent the destruction of the beneficial compounds. Replace ordinary garlic bread with herb butter, with bread spread with crushed garlic and cooked in the oven until golden, for the health benefits of garlic, without the saturated fats.

To combat the smell of garlic on the breath, chew a sprig of parsley. Some chefs claim that you can avoid suffering from 'garlic-breath' by removing the yellow shoot in the middle of each bulb.

Ginger zinger

Chew raw ginger root to relieve nausea associated with stomach upsets, travel sickness, migraine and pregnancy. Though in the case of morning sickness, it's recommended that no more than one gram a day should be taken. To prevent travel sickness, eat ginger half an hour before your journey.

Ginger stimulates digestion and prevent indigestion, bloating and gas. It also soothes stomach ache and pain associated with diarrhea and may reduce the risk of stomach ulcers.

It also seems to block the effects of prostaglandins – substances that can cause inflammation of blood vessels in the brain and lead to migraine. So it not only eases the nausea associated with migraines, but may also help stop the pain. Its anti-inflammatory properties also appear to ease muscular aches and pains due to heavy exercise, and menstrual cramps.

To relieve menstrual pain, or cold and flu symptoms, try a cup of hot ginger tea, made by pouring boiling water over 3 or 4 thin slices of ginger root and sweetened to taste, preferably with honey.

Anti-clotting properties, similar to those of aspirin, have been attributed to ginger. It boosts the circulation and lowers blood pressure and cholesterol, so it may help to prevent heart attacks and strokes.

To benefit from ginger's multiple health-giving properties and enjoy it's piquant flavor, use it in stir-fries, curries, cakes and cookies (biscuits). According to a Danish study in 1992, adding around one teaspoon (5mg) of powdered ginger or fresh ginger root to food daily helps to ease the pain of osteoarthritis and rheumatoid arthritis.

Horseradish help

Horseradish is a member of the cruciferous family, which includes broccoli and Brussels sprouts and like mustard, a close relation (see below), it contains glucosinolates. In fact horseradish supplies up to ten times more of these beneficial compounds than broccoli. The pungent root, which is used to make the spicy sauce that is traditionally served with roast beef, is rich in calcium, iron and magnesium, as well as B vitamins. It's also a good source of vitamin C – one tablepoon (15ml) of horseradish sauce supplies around one third of an adult's recommended daily intake.

Eating horseradish is thought to stimulate the digestive system. Herbalists recommend it for colds and flu because it clears the nasal passages. It helps to thin out mucus and has a natural antibiotic effect, making it useful in the prevention and treatment of sinusitis.

Must-have mustard

Mustard seeds contain plant nutrients called glucosinolates and enzymes that break these down into isothiocyanates (plant chemicals containing sulfur), which animal studies suggest prevent gastrointestinal and colorectal cancers. White mustard seeds are used to make yellow mustard, whilst the brown are used to make the Dijon variety.

By stimulating saliva production, mustard increases the appetite and aids digestion. It soothes upset stomachs, though too much can irritate. It's antiseptic, stimulates the circulation and is a good source of minerals, particularly selenium, magnesium, iron and zinc.

QUICK T!P
NUTMEG FOR NAUSEA
Nutmeg is rumored to ease nausea, flatulence and vomiting. It can also calm diarrhea. It's claimed to clear up eczema, when applied as a paste made by mixing ground nutmeg with water. It's great in savory dishes such as omelettes and cheese sauces, as well as desserts.

Paprika pick-me-up

Paprika is made from dried, red, mild to medium hot peppers. Like cayenne pepper, it contains capsaicin, and offers the same health benefits. It's sweeter and milder than cayenne.

Turmeric tonic

Turmeric is the spice that gives curry powder its yellow color. Its key health-boosting component is curcumin, which has anti-inflammatory properties. Studies suggest this compound may help prevent Alzheimer's and joint inflammation, as well as reduce cholesterol and hinder the progress of liver disease. Research at Reading University in the UK concluded it can help to ease abdominal pain and reduce diarrhea attacks in IBS sufferers. Evidence suggests that turmeric may have anti-cancer properties – particularly against bowel, colon and rectal cancers. To relieve eczema make a paste by simmering 30g (6 tsp) of turmeric powder in 150ml water until thickened. Store in the fridge and apply daily to affected areas, before covering with gauze.

Vanilla chiller

Vanilla is said to have a calming effect. It is also thought to aid digestion and act as an aphrodisiac and enhances the flavor of cakes and desserts. Use dried vanilla pods or pure vanilla extract, as opposed to vanilla flavoring. For a relaxing and comforting room spray combine 5 ml (1 tsp) of vanilla essence with 40 ml (8 tsps) of water in an atomizer.

Value vinegar

Vinegar can be a valuable addition to your diet, helping you to manage your weight and prevent osteoporosis and diabetes. Studies show that adding vinegar to food helps you to feel full for longer and therefore eat less.

Add a splash of ordinary malt, balsamic or white wine vinegar, or a vinaigrette dressing to dark leafy green vegetables – the acetic acid aids calcium absorption.

Vinegar seems to stabilize blood sugar levels by slowing down the absorption of glucose from food. It can benefit those with type 2 diabetes by helping to prevent the blood sugar rising too high after a meal. Evidence suggests that vinegar may even help prevent the development of type 2 diabetes, though further research is needed to confirm this.

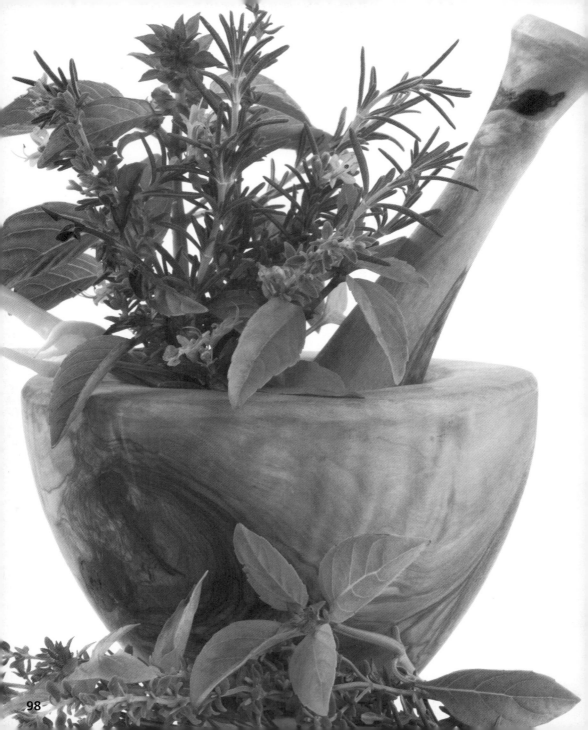

Healing Herbs

“ Herbs are the friend of the physician and the pride of cooks. **”**

Charlemagne

Chapter 6
Healing Herbs

Many of us keep herbs in our food cupboard to add flavor and interest to meals, but did you know studies confirm that ancient claims regarding their health-giving and medicinal properties are more than just folklore?

Many herbs contain even higher concentrations of antioxidants than fruit and vegetables and have anti-bacterial properties. They also contain phytochemicals (plant chemicals) and vitamins. Whilst we tend to consume herbs in much smaller amounts, they nevertheless offer a tasty way to improve our health.

Fresh herbs contain the most beneficial compounds, but if these are unavailable, dried herbs are still a valuable addition to your diet. They can be added to dishes as a healthy alternative to salt, and to enhance flavor. Some herbs make pleasant-tasting infusions (teas).

QUICK T!P
EASY HERBAL INFUSION
Use 10g (2 tsp) of fresh herbs, or 5g (1 tsp) of dried herbs per cup of boiling water. Place in a coffee cafetiere then add the boiling water. Replace the lid and leave to stand for five to ten minutes. Press down the plunger and pour. Sweeten with honey to taste. Drink whilst hot.

Growing your own herbs is easy. You can buy growing herbs from the fruit and vegetable section at your supermarket quite cheaply. Simply re-pot and place on a windowsill, or patio. Water and feed regularly.

Basil booster

Basil contains various flavonoids including orientin and vicenin, which have been shown to protect cells from radiation and to have antioxidant properties. It also contains volatile oils with antibacterial properties, helping to prevent some of the tummy bugs that cause diarrhea. Another volatile oil found in Basil, eugenol, has anti-inflammatory properties similar to those found in aspirin, making it beneficial to those with arthritis and other inflammatory conditions. Basil is believed to beat depression and ease cold symptoms too. Use it to add flavor to pastas and vegetable juices.

QUICK T!P
KEEP FLU AT BAY
Bay leaves contain traces of iron and phosphorous. They promote digestion and ease indigestion. They can ease flu symptoms by promoting sweating, when drunk as an infusion. The leaves are versatile, adding depth to savory dishes, such as soups, stew and casseroles and enhancing the flavor of rice pudding.

Coriander cure

Coriander appears to ease indigestion, bloating and diarrhoea as well as protect against food poisoning. Coriander seeds have a laxative effect. When crushed they can soothe mouth ulcers. Coriander also stimulates the appetite and helps to control the blood sugar. Research suggests it may help prevent colon cancer.

Colic relief

Dill soothes colic, easing gripe pains and dispersing flatulence. It's a common ingredient in commercial gripe waters, but you can make your own by adding one teaspoon (5g) of dill seeds to half a pint (500ml) of boiling water. Allow to cool and then strain. It's also antibacterial and acts as a diuretic.

Fen-tastic

In a recent two month trial fennel reduced period pain in young women. It may also stimulate milk production in lactating mothers. Both the plant and seeds help relieve indigestion and flatulence. It's also a diuretic. A tea made from the crushed seeds is recommended for relief from cystitis and kidney stones. Fennel tea also eases coughs, bronchitis and blocked sinuses. Fennel can be eaten raw and finely sliced, in salads, or roasted in olive oil as a tasty accompaniment to chicken. It's best to remove the tough outer layer first. Fennel isn't recommended for anyone at risk of seizures.

Lemon balm calm

Melissa officianalis, more commonly known as lemon balm, due to its nettle-like lemon-scented leaves, has long been used as a mood enhancer, because of its soothing and calming properties. It's said to ease tension and irritability and associated headaches and insomnia, as well as reduce hyperactivity. It's also believed to boost memory by making brain cells more receptive to acetylcholine, a brain chemical linked to memory. The leaves can be chopped and added to fish or meat dishes, as well as drunk as a refreshing infusion. Or blend them into a melon or pear smoothie, to enhance the flavor.

Anti-aging oregano

Also known as marjoram, weight for weight, oregano contains up to 20 times more antioxidants than other herbs, and up to four times more than blueberries.

When drunk as an infusion it's thought to relieve cold and flu symptoms. The oregano herb is safe to use during pregnancy, but oregano volatile oil isn't, as it may harm the baby.

Pick parsley for PMS

Parsley is particularly good for women. Its diuretic properties are thought to relieve the water retention associated with periods. It may also help to normalize menstrual flow and relieve cramps and PMS. Taken daily, the phytoestrogens it contains can ease menopausal symptoms. It contains iron to help prevent anemia. Other minerals such as calcium, magnesium and potassium act as a general tonic. It's also a source of Vitamin C. Drinking a parsley infusion is reported to relieve cystitis. Chewing parsley freshens the breath. Other suggested uses include as a poultice for acne, eczema, bites, stings and sore eyes. It goes well with fish, or vegetable dishes or juices.

Peppermint pep-up

Peppermint stimulates the mind and helps clear headaches. It's very effective as a digestive aid, easing indigestion and flatulence and is good for IBS sufferers, as it eases gut spasms. When drunk as an infusion it relieves cold and flu symptoms, clearing blocked nasal passages and promoting sweating. Animal studies suggest it may also protect against cancers of the skin, colon and lungs. Herbalists claim it can both prevent and relieve asthma symptoms. It can be added to salad dressings, savory sauces and even desserts. In hot weather, blend mint leaves into your smoothies, to make them more refreshing and cooling.

Rosemary relief

Seven grammes – just over a teaspoon – of rosemary contains as many antioxidants as 55g of blueberries. It has antiseptic properties and stimulates digestion. It also freshens the breath. It's thought to boost the circulation to the brain, helping to protect it from aging and Alzheimer's, as well as improve memory and mood. For a headache cure, or relief from cold symptoms, drink an infusion made from the spikes.

Wise up to sage

Sage is recommended as a memory enhancer and may also help prevent Alzheimer's. Research suggests the herb inhibits enzymes, which attack acetylcholine, a chemical involved in learning and memory. It's also recommended for women suffering from hot flashes, both during and after the menopause. It may reduce flashes by regulating hypothalamus function. It can be added to stews and casseroles, omelettes and scrambled eggs, or drunk as a tea. It's not recommended for breastfeeding women, as it may reduce milk flow.

Tarragon tranquility

Tarragon has calming, sedative properties and tarragon tea is said to promote sleep. It also stimulates the appetite and aids digestion. It can promote or increase menstrual flow, so should be avoided in pregnancy. It's commonly added to fish dishes.

Take thyme

Thyme is antibacterial and when drunk as an infusion can relieve cystitis, ease chest congestion from colds and treat chronic coughs. It's also good for digestion and stimulates the circulation.

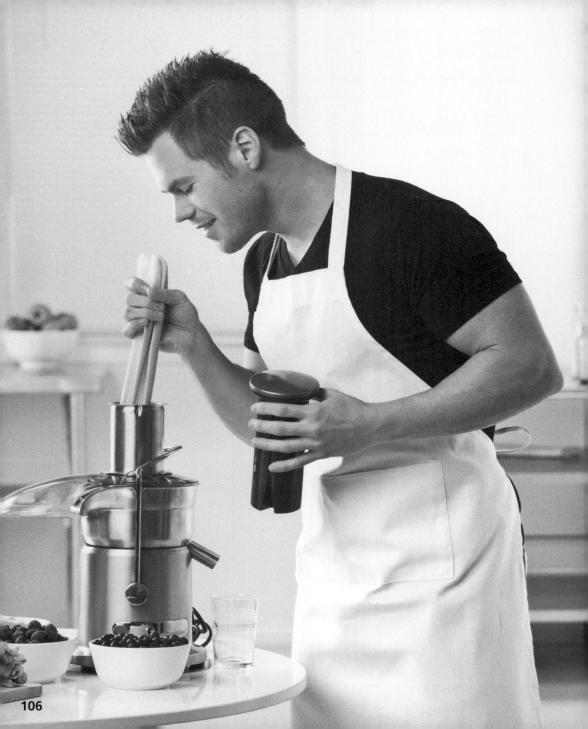

Healthy Quenchers

“ The core beverage we need for life for health? It's water. **”**

Barry Popkin

Chapter 7
Healthy Quenchers

Ensuring you drink adequate amounts of fluid is essential for good health. The body is around 70 percent water. We can go without food for around five weeks, but can only last about five days without fluids. Our cells, tissues, organs and body processes all require water. You need around six to eight 225ml – 8oz glasses of liquid daily. But this can vary according to your age, gender, activity levels and the temperature. Fruit and vegetables, with their high water content, will also hydrate you. Let your thirst guide you. Straw-colored, odorless urine indicates you're getting enough fluids. Dark colored, strong-smelling urine suggests you need to drink more water. Sugary drinks provide empty calories, and can lead to weight gain, as well as tooth decay, so are best avoided. Some drinks can deliver particular health benefits, though in the case of tea, coffee and alcohol, moderation is usually advised.

Water baby

Drinking between one and a half and two liters of water each day is one of the easiest steps you can take to improve your health. Have a glass each morning, a glass between and with meals and a glass at your bedside at night. Experts claim that being well-hydrated reduces the risk of obesity, constipation, kidney stones and urinary tract and breast cancers, as well as preventing headaches and tiredness.

Ice is nice

Drinking water ice cold has been shown to boost the metabolism, because the body needs to heat it up before using it. Plain, still, water is viewed as the healthiest choice. To make it even more refreshing, try adding a few sprigs of mint, or basil, or slices of cucumber, lime, or lemon.

QUICK T!P
MILK MAID
A recent study concluded that drinking 500ml (1 pint) of milk daily more than halves the risk of insulin resistance (where the body doesn't respond properly to insulin), which can cause heart disease, stroke and type 2 diabetes. Other research suggests that milk rehydrates the body after exercise for longer than expensive sports drinks, because it's removed from the body more slowly, due to the protein, fat, and sugar it contains. Milk also contains vitamins and minerals, including bone-building calcium, and it doesn't cause tooth decay. The calcium in milk and dairy foods has been shown to help reduce PMS. Go for skim (skimmed), reduced-fat (semi-skimmed), or low-fat (1 percent fat) milk, as they contain less saturated fat than whole milk.

Just juicing

Juicing is another way of ensuring you benefit from fruit and vegetables. Enthusiasts claim that juicing releases the nutrients that are stored in the fiber of the whole fruit or vegetable, so that they can be absorbed, rather than expelled with the fiber.

QUICK T!P
DRINK ORANGE JUICE
A glass of orange juice each day provides approximately 60mg of immunity-boosting vitamin C and folic acid, which helps prevent birth defects. If drunk with meals, it also increases iron absorption.

Avoid asthma with apple juice

Recent research suggests that children who drink apple juice at least once a day are less likely to develop asthma. Juices from concentrate work just as well as fresh. Natural chemicals in the apples, such as flavonoids and phenolic acids seem to have an anti-inflammatory effect on the airways, preventing wheezing. Children don't appear to gain the same benefits from eating apples themselves – yet studies have shown that adults do.

Smooth operator

Fruit smoothies are a great way to get your daily fruit quota. Because you're blending, rather than juicing, you get the benefits of the whole fruit, including the fiber. This easy, energy-boosting recipe for two, uses natural yogurt, banana and honey. Add any fruit you like.

1 large banana

2-3 handfuls of fruit

285ml (/½ pint) unsweetened natural yogurt

Runny honey (optional)

Cinnamon, or nutmeg (optional)

Place the banana and your chosen fruit into a blender. Blend for 30 seconds. Add the natural yogurt, and honey to taste. Blend again to a milk-shake consistency. Sprinkle with cinnamon or nutmeg and serve.

Stop for tea

Drinking tea – ordinary black, or green, or white oolong, provides an array of health benefits. Tea contains flavonoids, catechins and polyphenols – powerful antioxidants, believed to prevent heart disease and cancer. Green tea contains the most, followed by oolong and black teas. Tea also appears promote normal blood pressure, by increasing the elasticity of arteries. But some research suggests that adding milk to tea blocks this effect.

Green tea is thought to assist weight loss by promoting the release of the hormone norepinephrine which curbs the appetite. It also contains polyphenols which raise the metabolic rate and encourage fat burning. Evidence suggests that all three teas – including ordinary black tea may also protect against stroke, osteoporosis and bacterial and viral infections. Furthermore, your daily cup of tea (cuppa) is anti-inflammatory and helps protect against allergies. Jigging the tea bag up and down a few times releases more of the beneficial antioxidants.

Despite recent claims to the contrary, it seems that tea is hydrating, provided you drink no more than six cups of average strength daily. This would give you a caffeine intake of around 300mg, which shouldn't have a strong diuretic effect.

Tea helps you relax, because it contains a substance called theanine, which is believed to act as a tranquilizer, without affecting concentration. Recent tests showed that when tea drinkers are exposed to stress, their levels of the stress hormone cortisol drop much more quickly than those of non-tea drinkers.

Your dental health can benefit from drinking tea too. The fluoride it contains strengthens tooth enamel. It also appears to prevent the growth of oral bacteria linked to bad breath and tooth decay.

Tea boosts insulin activity, helping to maintain a steady blood sugar, which helps to keep the appetite in check.

It's best to avoid drinking tea with a meal. Try to wait half an hour, because it contains tannins, which prevent your body from absorbing iron from non-meat sources, such as wholegrains, peas or dried fruit. Tea also contains polyphenols which bind with iron, making absorption more difficult. Drinking your tea with a slice of lemon may help, because its vitamin C content aids iron absorption.

Redbush or Rooibos tea is lower in tannin than regular tea. It's also caffeine- free, so it's good to drink at bed-time, if caffeine tends to keep you awake.

QUICK T!P

HERBAL TEAS

Herbal teas make a refreshing alternative to tea and coffee and provide the health-boosting properties of the herbs or spices they contain. Choose from a vast array, ranging from the old favorites, ginger, peppermint and chamomile, to more exotic blends containing vanilla, or ginseng. Or make your own using fresh herbs – see Chapter 6 – Healing Herbs.

Coffee cure

Most people know that a cup of coffee can increase mental alertness and concentration and counteract the effects of tiredness and fatigue. But did you know that coffee may have other health benefits?

A long-term study indicated that drinking three cups of coffee a day can reduce the risk of mental decline in old age and cut the risk of Alzheimer's by half. The elderly have higher levels of adenosine, a brain chemical that weakens gamma rhythms, which are involved in memory and learning processes. The caffeine in coffee appears to reduce the risk of memory loss and Alzheimer's by blocking the effects of adenosine. Coffee may also reduce the risk of Parkinson's disease, gallstones and rectal cancer. A US study claimed that drinking four cups of coffee daily could reduce the incidence of gout in men.

Coffee can also help to relieve headaches, when drunk at the same time as taking painkillers such as ibuprofen. The caffeine content increases the painkilling effect, by improving absorption. A strong cup of coffee can abort a migraine, which can occur when blood vessels in the head dilate. The caffeine constricts the blood vessels, relieving the painful symptoms of blood vessel dilation.

According to the Australian Institute of Sport, a cup of strong black coffee 1-2 hours before exercise stimulates the release of fats into the blood stream, which allows the body to burn fat as its main energy source, thus speeding up fat loss. Another study suggests that drinking coffee and being active can inhibit skin cancer.

Coffee quota

But, as always, moderation is the best policy. Drinking more than 4-5 cups of coffee daily might cause health problems. The caffeine in coffee is addictive and can cause anxiety, insomnia, tremors and an irregular heartbeat. Women who drink eight or more cups of coffee a day during pregnancy appear more likely to suffer a miscarriage or stillbirth. Heavy coffee drinkers also seem to be more at risk of heart disease, osteoporosis and arthritis.

QUICK T!P

LOWER-CAL COFFEE
Be careful how you take your coffee. A large latte made with whole milk can contain around 18g (½oz) of saturated fat – nearly the recommended daily amount. A cappuccino is slightly better, with around a third of the amount of saturated fat. Ask for 'skinny' versions made with skim (skimmed), reduced-fat (semi-skimmed), or low-fat (1 percent fat) milk, to reduce the saturated fat and calories. Or go for expresso. Avoid adding sugar and syrups, or topping it with whipped cream, chocolate or caramel. Cinnamon is a healthier choice.

You should cocoa!

Cocoa contains flavonols which appear to boost brain-power and reduce the risk of vascular dementia – caused by blood-flow problems to the brain, stroke, CHD, cancer and diabetes.

One particular flavonol, epicatechin, is believed to improve circulation, boosting blood flow to the brain and improving cardiovascular health. It also helps keep blood sugar levels stable.

Avoid drinking chocolate drinks which contain added sugar, salt and flavorings. Opt for pure cocoa to gain the most benefits.

Enjoy a tipple

Enjoying a tipple could help you to manage your weight and boost your health. A glass of red wine such as Pinot Noir, Cabernet Sauvignon or Merlot, not only provides the benefits attributed to grapes (see Chapter 4 – Superfoods), but also others linked with alcohol. These include increased HDL or 'good cholesterol' and decreased fibrinogen, the body's blood clotting agent, which reduces the risk of heart disease and stroke. Recent research in Portugal suggested that red wine might help to control weight; it's thought it raises estrogen levels, which cuts the amount of fat stored in the body. Another study in the US claimed that women who drink wine – especially red wine – in moderation are less likely to gain weight than those who drink soft drinks. It's thought that this is because any excess energy from alcohol is burned off as heat, rather than stored as fat.

Alcohol is also thought to offer protection against Alzheimer's, colds and flu. All wine seems to improve lung health, but white has the most effect. It's thought that antioxidants in white wines mop up toxins in the blood and reduce inflammation in the airways.

But don't binge

But remember, moderation is the key! More than 3 units daily/ 14 units weekly for women and 4 units daily/21 units weekly for men, can have a detrimental effect on health. On average, one small glass of red wine contains 1.5 units of alcohol. A large glass typically contains 2 units.

Binge drinking, which is classified as drinking more than double the recommended daily amount in one go, appears to not only increase the risk of breast cancer in women, but to also stimulate tumor growth. It may raise the risk of bowel cancer too and is linked to cirrhosis of the liver. In both men and women, it can raise the risk of obesity, because alcohol contains 7 calories per gram. Heavy drinking is also associated with high blood pressure, which increases your chances of suffering from strokes and heart attacks.

Pregnant women are advised not to drink alcohol at all. Alcohol crosses the placenta and enters the baby's bloodstream. It can damage developing organs and prevent normal growth and development.

Sip slimline

Between ten and twenty percent of your daily calorie intake can come from drinks. Sugar-sweetened beverages, sugary drinks, drinks with cream or full-fat milk and sweet alcoholic drinks are the main culprits. Try these changes – they're painless, and you could soon be slimmer and healthier:

- Gradually reduce the amount of sugar you add to tea and coffee, then cut it out altogether

- Swap sugary drinks such as coke and lemonade for sugar-free versions or, better still, water. A person who drinks 500ml of coke or lemonade each day, would lose 25 pounds in weight each year, simply by making this switch!

- Avoid fruit juice drinks, which are high in sugar – opt for unsweetened fruit juice instead

- Dilute unsweetened fruit juice with water

- Swap regular fruit drink (squash) for sugar-free fruit drink

- Choose drinks made with skim (skimmed), reduced-fat (semi-skimmed), or low-fat (1 percent fat) milk, instead of full-fat. Better still, drink tea and coffee without milk if you can

- Cut your intake of sweet or creamy drinks by swapping short, fat glasses and mugs for tall thin glasses and mugs – you'll automatically drink less

- Drink skim (skimmed), reduced-fat (semi-skimmed) or low-fat (1 percent fat) milk, rather than full-fat

- Alternate drinking alcohol with sugar-free soft drinks, or water

- Choose sugar-free mixers, such as diet coke

- Drink wine spritzer, which is wine mixed with soda, instead of wine

- Choose dry versions of alcoholic drinks – such as dry white wine – they contain less sugar

- Replace sugary alcopops with a shot of spirit and a low-calorie mixer

- Swap a gin and tonic, containing 93 calories, for a gin and slimline tonic, which contains only 53 calories

- Avoid drinking more than one or two low-alcohol or 'lite' beers or lagers daily, as they can be higher in calories than regular versions

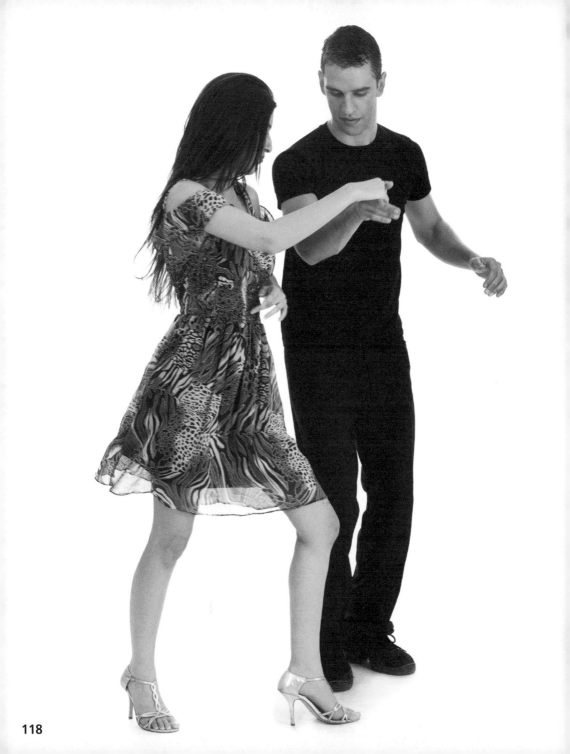

No Time For The Gym?

“ Whenever I feel like exercise, I lie down until the feeling passes. **”**

Robert Hutchins

Chapter 8
No Time For The Gym?

Physical activity helps you to lose weight by burning calories and boosting the metabolism. It can also reduce the risk of heart disease, type 2 diabetes, some cancers, osteoporosis, dementia and Alzheimer's.

Apart from changes in diet, the other major factor in today's rapidly increasing obesity rates is the decrease in physical activity levels, due to the vast changes in lifestyles over the past few decades. Our parents and grandparents didn't go to the gym, but they were much slimmer and fitter, because their everyday lives involved far more activity.

The steep rise in car ownership and public transport means fewer people walk or cycle on a daily basis. Increased use of labor-saving domestic appliances and devices has reduced the amount of physical activity involved in running a home.

The current recommendations for adults are that they should participate in moderate intensity exercise, such as walking, for at least 30 minutes, for five or more days a week. For weight loss and management, aim at 60 minutes for at least five days a week. If you have an inactive lifestyle, it's best to build up gradually to these levels. For example, you could begin by walking ten minutes daily, before increasing to fifteen minutes and then thirty minutes. Eventually you could aim at two thirty minute walks daily.

Research suggests that the best way to achieve fitness is to incorporate physical activity into your daily routine, just as our forebears did, rather than joining the gym; huge sums of money are wasted on unused gym memberships each year, with people citing lack of time and boredom as the main reasons for their non-attendance. This chapter shows how small lifestyle changes can have a big effect on your weight and fitness.

Little and often

Being active several times a day benefits your metabolism more than just doing one long bout of exercise. This is because during physical activity your metabolic rate increases and doesn't go back to normal for up to two hours – depending on the intensity.

Make a stand

If you stand, rather than sit, you'll burn an extra 70 calories an hour. If you stood for 20 minutes a day, six days a week, you would burn off 2lbs of fat in a year!

Leg it

Fit more walking into your daily routine. Walking is an aerobic exercise which increases cardiovascular fitness and lowers blood pressure, cholesterol and body fat, thus reducing the risk of strokes and heart attacks. Recent research reveals that whereas high intensity activity, such as a gym workout, tends to burn more carbohydrate than fat, moderate intensity exercise, like walking, burns more fat than carbohydrate. Other benefits include improved mental health, reduced risk of type 2 diabetes, breast and colon cancers and stronger bones and muscles. Park your car further from the office, or the shops. Get off the bus or train one stop earlier.

Walk away weight

Walking also aids weight control. Research suggests that women on average take 5,000 steps daily and men 6,000. Overweight people take on average 1,500 to 2,000 fewer steps daily than those within a healthy weight range. So if you need to lose weight, try walking an extra 2,000 steps a day – roughly the equivalent of fifteen minutes of walking – and you'll burn around 450 calories a week. Even if you made no other changes in your lifestyle, in a year you would burn off around 3kg (6lbs) in weight. Fit in a 15 minute walk during your lunch break, instead of sitting at your desk. At weekends follow the tips below to fit more walking into your routine. Gradually increase your walking pace. The faster you walk the more steps you'll clock up. Seven thousand steps daily have been shown to improve fitness, but 10,000 can increase fitness even more dramatically and result in faster weight loss. A pedometer is cheap to buy and a useful tool to help you determine whether you need to fit more walking into your daily routine.

QUICK T!P

WALKIES!
A recent survey indicated that dog owners actually take more exercise and are fitter than gym members. On average a dog walker clocks up 676 miles each year compared to only 468 miles for a gym-goer. Dog walkers have slightly lower blood pressure and their heart rates return to their resting rate more quickly than gym users. The average resting heart rate of dog walkers is generally lower than that of gym users. Dog owners tend to take more exercise because they have to exercise their pets 'come rain or shine'. So, if you want to enjoy the benefits of your own canine personal fitness trainer, buy a dog, or offer to walk a neighbor's!

Be a domestic god/goddess

Household chores such as vacuuming, dusting and cleaning, tone arm and leg muscles and increase the heart rate, making housework a good all-round cardiovascular exercise. Mopping, dusting, cleaning and vacuuming burn around 250 calories per hour, so doing housework can help you to control your weight. Work to the beat of your favorite CD to make cleaning more fun! Ironing burns around 140 calories per hour. If you press down firmly, you can give your arm muscles a good workout. Research suggests that if you approach housework as if you're doing a gym workout, you're more likely to lose weight! As you get fitter, you can speed up your domestic routine to burn off even more calories.

Clean your own windows!

Clean your own windows and you'll not only save money, but also give your whole body a workout. Climbing up the ladders tones the leg muscles, whilst wiping firms the upper arms.

Peg it

Peg out clothes on the washing line instead of tumble-drying and it's not just the environment and your energy bills that'll benefit. As you reach up, your whole body gets a good stretch and carrying a full laundry basket outdoors works your arm muscles.

QUICK T!P

DITCH THE REMOTE
Throwing away the remote control will help you burn off around 1kg (2 lbs) in weight in a year.

Walkie-talkie

Use a cordless or mobile phone and walk around the house as you talk.

Take TV breaks

Rather than sitting in front of the TV all evening, get up and walk around during the ad breaks, or in between programmes. You could even fit in a chore, like emptying the trash (rubbish) or washing dishes. In three hours of viewing you could clock up as much as forty five minutes of activity!

Green gym

Thirty minutes of gardening can offer the same benefits as a workout, especially if it includes digging. Even light gardening tasks can improve strength and agility.

General garden chores such as weeding, mowing and digging burn between 200 and 500 calories per hour and strengthen and tone various muscles. Use a manual mower rather than an electrical one. Use a watering can, rather than a garden hose, to give your arm muscles a workout.

Gardening is also a weight-bearing exercise deemed more effective than jogging for strengthening bones. Sunlight on the skin stimulates the production of vitamin D, which helps the body to absorb bone-strengthening calcium, making gardening excellent protection against osteoporosis.

Wash the car by hand

Wash the car by hand, instead of going to the car wash.

Leave the car

For short trips, such as popping to the grocery store, leave the car at home and walk.

Stop the school run

If your children's school is within walking distance ditch the school run and walk them to school instead.

Family fitness

Too busy looking after your children to exercise? Pushing a stroller (pram) or buggy around the park is good exercise for you and provides fresh air and a change of scenery for baby. Play ball games with older children. Take them for a long walk, or visit your local swimming baths.

Pace the platform

If your train is late, walk up and down the platform, rather than standing still. You can do the same at the bus stop.

" If it weren't for the fact that the TV and the fridge were so far apart, some of us wouldn't get any exercise at all. **"**

Joey Adams

Supermarket shape-up

Use a basket, rather than a cart (trolley), when you only need a few groceries and you'll strengthen and tone your shoulder and arm muscles.

Leave the elevator (lift)

Taking the stairs instead of the elevator (lift) will work your cardiovascular system, increase your level of fitness, tone your leg and thigh muscles and burn calories. If you drive, park your car at the top of the multistorey parking lot (car park) and use the stairs.

Walk the escalator

Walking both up and down escalators helps to tone the bottom and burn calories!

Get active at the office

Leave your desk and walk around regularly. Even just a couple of minutes of activity every hour will equal one and a quarter hours of activity each working week. Walk to your colleagues' desks to pass on information instead of emailing. Walk to the water dispenser every hour for a refill and you'll boost your hydration and your activity levels. Make trips to the kitchen to make drinks.

Desk-ercises to beat DVT

Sitting at a desk for long periods poses the same risk of deep-vein thrombosis as air travel does. It's important not to sit still for periods of longer than an hour. The following exercises can help.

- Clench your calf and thigh muscles several times each hour

- With your legs stretched out in front of you, raise your feet and hold for one minute

- Sit with your feet directly in line with your knees. Raise your feet and hold for one minute

Desk-stretches

Sitting at a desk whilst looking at a computer screen and using a keyboard for long periods can cause muscular pain and discomfort in the neck, shoulders, back, arms and hands. Stretching eases muscular tension, whilst increasing flexibility and reducing stress.

Aim at doing 2 or 3 stretches, every one or two hours, and notice the difference at the end of the working day.

Neck stretch – Sit up straight, with your shoulders relaxed. Looking straight ahead, try to touch your left shoulder with your left ear. Hold for 5 seconds. Return head upright. Repeat on each side up to five times.

Shoulder rotation – Sitting upright, rotate each shoulder alternately 2 or 3 times – first forwards and then backwards.

Back arch – Sitting upright, place both hands on your lower back. Arch your back by pushing your hips forward and pulling your shoulders back. Hold for 10 seconds and repeat up to three times.

Arm stretch – Stretch both arms out in front of you at shoulder height, palms upright. Bend forearms back and touch shoulders with fingertips. Repeat up to five times.

Hand stretch – Clench your fists tightly for 5 seconds, then extend your fingers. Relax. Repeat up to five times.

Be a disco diva

Dancing is an enjoyable way to get fit that can be combined with a healthy social life. It offers numerous emotional, physical and mental health benefits, including increased cardiovascular fitness, stronger bones and muscles, better co-ordination, agility and flexibility, and improved balance and spatial awareness. One hour on the dance floor enables the average person to burn off 200 calories upwards – depending on the type of dancing. Strutting your stuff on the dance floor also improves your mental well-being, wards off dementia and develops social skills.

Laugh yourself lean

Research suggests that laughing each day for about fifteen minutes burns as much energy as walking for half an hour, gives muscles a workout and raises the heart rate. You could lose up to 5lbs (2kg) in weight in a year. So if you want to improve your figure and fitness the easy way, dig out those comedy videos and joke books and get giggling!

Fidget away fat

Scientists at the Mayo Clinic in Minnesota found that one of the biggest factors affecting a person's weight is their level of Non-Exercise Activity Thermogenesis – NEAT – more commonly known as fidgeting! They found that slim people tend to fidget more than overweight people and as a result burn up to 350 calories a day more.

If you're not a fidget, try to become one! Change position more often when standing or sitting. Tap your feet when seated. Pace up and down whilst waiting for the kettle to boil.

Temperature control

Turn down the thermostat at home and at the office and your body will burn fat to keep warm. Experts believe you can burn up to 250 calories a day trying to maintain a comfortable body temperature.

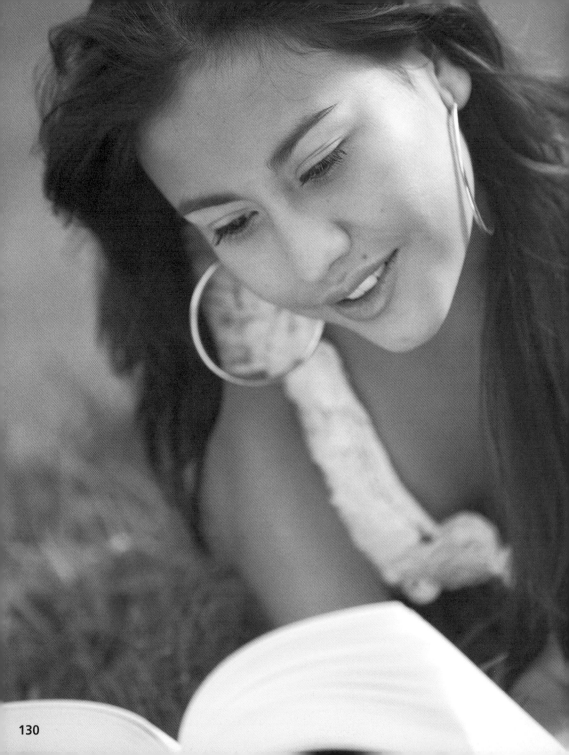

Stress Busters

" To the mind that is still, the whole universe surrenders. **"**

Lao Tzu

Chapter 9
Stress Busters

Stress is how our mind and body react to responsibility or pressure which leaves us feeling inadequate or unable to cope. It depends on our perception of a situation and our ability to deal with it. A situation one person finds stressful, another may not. A recent study at the California University in San Francisco and Minnesota University involving 121 women found that sticking to just 1,200 calories a day raised stress levels – another argument against following a strict diet and supporting focussing on eating healthily instead.

The brain responds to stress by preparing our body to either stay and face up to the perceived threat, or to run away. This involves the release of hormones including adrenaline, noradrenaline and cortisol into the bloodstream. As a result the heart-rate and breathing patterns speed up and we might sweat. Glucose and fatty acid levels in the blood increase to give us the energy to deal with the threat. This is commonly known as the 'fight or flight' response.

Studies suggest that, over a prolonged period, these chemical effects of stress can be detrimental to health, leading to an increased risk of high blood pressure, CHD, stroke, cancer, obesity, diabetes, depression and even memory loss and fertility problems.

If the cause of stress is not removed or controlled, cortisol levels remain high. The body then adapts to this constant state of emergency by increasing the appetite for high-energy sugary or fatty foods and keeping a store of fat around the waist, near the vital organs, where it can be quickly converted back into energy. This is the most dangerous place to store fat because it's linked to an increased risk of coronary heart disease (CHD), stroke, and type 2 diabetes.

Bad habits

As well as overeating, we often deal with stress by adopting other unhealthy habits, such as smoking, and drinking too much alcohol, the ill-effects of which we are all aware.

With many of us living our lives at an increasingly fast pace and often under pressure to achieve and perform, stress has become a major cause of ill-health that is estimated to be responsible for 50 to 60 percent of lost working days.

Finding ways of dealing with stress is clearly essential for a long and happy life. The following tips may help.

Reduce overload

Overload is the feeling that you have too much to do, that you're juggling too many balls. It often happens gradually – you take on extra roles and duties without realizing that they're piling up. For example, you agree to extra responsibilities at work and then a family member falls ill and needs regular visits. As your commitments pile up, so do the feelings that you can't cope, along with your stress levels. The next five tips will help you to reduce overload in your life.

QUICK T!P

KEEP A STRESS JOURNAL
For a couple of weeks keep a record of situations, times, places and people that make you feel stressed. Once you've identified your stressors, find ways to avoid or minimise them.

Manage your time

If you constantly feel under pressure and stressed due to a lack of time you could look at how you use it. Keep a diary for a few days to see where your time goes and then see which activities you can cut out, or reduce, to make time for the things that are most important to you. If you commute, use the time positively, rather just gazing out of the window. For example, read a book, plan your diary, or relax, listening to your favorite music.

QUICK T!P
JUST SAY 'NO'

If you feel overburdened with chores and your stress levels are rising as a result, try saying ' no' to non-essential tasks you don't have time for or just don't want to do.

What a to do!

Make a 'To-Do' list to help prevent yourself from feeling overwhelmed by the tasks you need to do. Then prioritize, so that you do the most important and urgent jobs first. You'll feel more in control and organized. You won't forget to do something that's important or miss a deadline. 'To Do' lists work well both at work and at home, helping you to be more efficient and less stressed.

Learn to delegate

Overload often happens when you convince yourself that no one else can meet your high standards, so it's easier if you do everything yourself. This inevitably leads to physical and mental overload. The solution is to accept that you can't know and do everything, so you need to learn to listen to other people's ideas and opinions and to delegate. Ask your partner and children to help with tasks around the home and garden. Accept offers of help at work.

Think positive

Affirmations are positive statements you make about and to yourself, which help raise your self esteem. The higher your self-esteem, the more able you will be to deal with life's challenges, and you'll be less likely to suffer from stress. Remember stress arises from your perception of a situation, rather than from the situation itself. If you find yourself in a situation which is causing you stress, visualize yourself coping with it and use an affirmation. For example, if you have a forthcoming job interview or exam which is worrying you, picture yourself performing well and use a positive affirmation such as 'I am capable of doing this job' or ' I can pass this exam'. This should increase your confidence in your ability to deal with the situation, and as a result it should become less stressful.

When something bad happens, instead of thinking about how terrible the situation is, look for the positive aspects of it, if you can. Try to find solutions to the problem, or change your perception of it, perhaps viewing it as an opportunity for personal growth. For example, being made redundant might seem like a very worrying and negative event at first but, if you decide to use it as an opportunity to retrain and start a new career doing something that you really enjoy, it can become a catalyst for positive change.

Live in the present

Mindfulness has been shown to reduce stress levels. It involves focussing on the here and now, rather than worrying about the past or future and has its roots in Buddhism. It's based on the philosophy that we can't change the past, or predict the future, but we can affect what's happening right now. By living fully in the present you can perform to the best of your ability, whereas worrying about the past and future can hamper how you function now, and increase stress levels unnecessarily.

QUICK T!P
CLEAR CLUTTER
Getting rid of unused items and tidying your home, or work space, helps you to feel in control, and this in turn leads to you feeling calmer.

Laugh a lot

Laughter really is the best medicine! Not only does it make you fitter, it also relieves stress and boosts the immune system. After a bout of laughter the levels of cortisol and other stress hormones in the body reduce. A good belly-laugh also relaxes the muscles in the upper body.

Pet therapy

Stroking your pet dog or cat lowers your blood pressure and reduces stress. Research indicates that the heart rate slows down and the body stops producing the stress hormones cortisol and adrenaline.

The sound of music

Listen to your favorite CD. Evidence suggests that taking time out to listen to music you enjoy reduces anxiety and may even relieve pain.

Chew gum

Chewing gum has been shown to reduce muscular tension and the effects of stress on the brain. Chewing appears to stimulate parts of the brain which have a role in lowering tension and may reduce the production of neurochemicals associated with stress.

Go back to nature

Go back to nature to reduce your stress levels. Activities such as looking at the sea, going for a walk in the park or the countryside, or even gardening, have proved to reduce heart rate, blood pressure and muscle tension.

Experts think that the higher levels of negative ions near areas with running water, trees and mountains may be partly responsible. Others link it to 'biophilia' – the idea that man has a natural affinity with nature. Research suggests that people living near green areas enjoy a longer lifespan and better health, than those who live in urban environments.

Walk away worries

Walking reduces stress by stimulating the production of endorphins – natural tranquilizers which give a feeling of well-being, reducing depression, anxiety and stress. As a result walkers feel more positive and more able to deal with problems, which leads to further reductions in stress levels.

Sunshine soother

Exposure to natural sunlight raises serotonin levels in the brain, boosting both mood and the ability to deal with stress. But make sure that you follow current advice regarding sunshine exposure:

- Stay in the shade from 11am-3pm

- Ensure you never burn

- Cover up

- Take extra care with children

- Use factor 15+ sunscreen

Social support

Research shows that people who have a good social network tend to enjoy better mental health than those who don't. So make time to see family and friends regularly.

Wind down at work …

Whilst too many interruptions in the form of emails, text messages, phone calls and colleagues chatting can cause the work to pile up and stress levels to rise, being sociable at work is a stress reducer. A chat with colleagues over a cup of tea (cuppa) and encouragement and support from your supervisor all help to keep you happy at work.

Plant power

Placing a plant on your desk can reduce your stress levels. Researchers believe they reduce levels of pollutants in the air and improve humidity. Also, nature has a calming effect on people.

QUICK T!P
SWITCH OFF!
To help you switch off, switch off your mobile phone or Blackberry outside of work and especially on vacation (holiday)!

Take a break

Try to schedule regular 'me-time' breaks into you daily routine. Even two fifteen-minute breaks during your working day, when you do whatever you want, can help to lower stress levels. Something as simple as having a cup of tea and a chat, or reading the newspaper, can have a positive effect as it can take your mind off your work situation.

Breathe deep

Deep breathing has been shown reduce the heart rate, relax muscles, release tension and boost mood. Next time you feel stressed, try this simple exercise. Inhale slowly to a count of five, allowing your tummy to expand, hold for a count of five and then breathe out slowly to a count of five, whilst slowly flattening your tummy. Repeat up to ten times.

Two-minute revitalizer

Every two or three hours try this two minute exercise to release tension and revive energy. Close your eyes then slowly massage your temples, gently but firmly, for one minute in an anti-clockwise direction and then for one minute clockwise. At the same time picture a relaxing scene e.g. lying on the beach on vacation (holiday) or relaxing in front of a big log fire with a glass of wine – whatever conjures up relaxation for you.

Light a candle

A lit candle has a calming, almost hypnotic effect. Focussing on a candle flame whilst practising deep breathing is a simple form of meditation.

Sniff lavender

Japanese researchers found that sniffing lavender oil for five minutes a day dramatically reduces the stress hormone cortisol. Rosemary oil was found to be equally effective.

Touch therapy

Massage is one of the oldest and most effective methods of counteracting stress. Daily tensions and stress can make us tense and lead to pain and muscle stiffness. The Greek philosopher Hippocrates – the 'father of medicine' recognized the value of massage, claiming it 'can loosen a joint that is too rigid'. Massage involves touch – a powerful tool that can ease away tensions, aches and pains. It works by stimulating the release of endorphins – the body's own painkillers and serotonin, a brain chemical associated with relaxation. It also decreases the level of stress hormones in the blood and improves blood circulation.

Make your own massage oil by mixing a few drops of your favorite aromatherapy oil e.g. lavender, chamomile or ylang ylang into a carrier oil, such as almond or grapeseed. The easiest way to enjoy the benefits of massage is for you and a partner to massage each other's back, neck and shoulders, using the basic techniques listed below:

Stroking/effleurage – glide both hands over the skin in rhythmic fanning or circular motions.

Kneading – using alternate hands, squeeze and release flesh between fingers and thumbs, as if you're kneading dough.

Friction – use your thumbs to apply even pressure to static points, or make small circles, on either side of the spine.

Hacking – relax your hands and use the sides quickly and alternately to give short, sharp taps all over.

Playing some relaxing music at the same time can enhance the feeling of relaxation.

Hand-y relaxer

Next time you're feeling stressed and tense use your thumbs to apply pressure to each of your solar plexus reflexes, which are in the middle of each palm, about two-thirds of the way up.

Meditate

Learn Transcendental Meditation – it's a simple technique which, if practised daily, has been shown to relieve stress and tiredness and increase energy and the ability to think clearly. To learn more go to www.tm.org

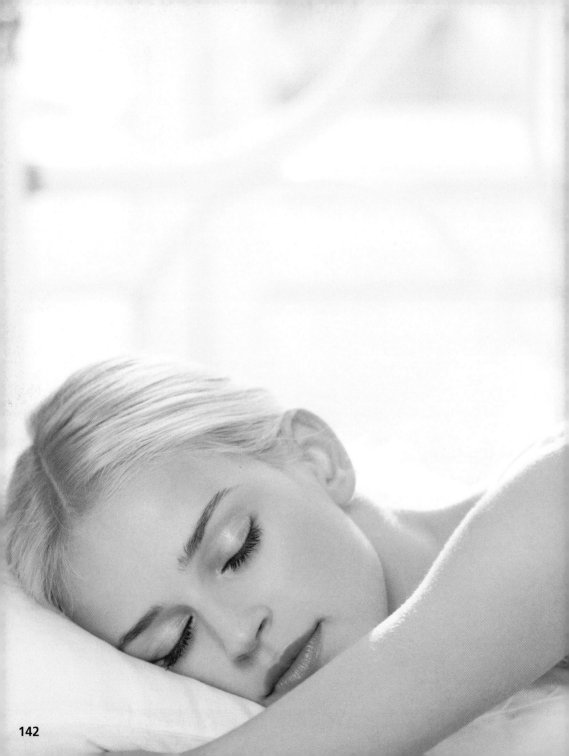

Sleep Tight

" Oh sleep!
it is a gentle thing.
Beloved from
pole to pole. **"**

Samuel Taylor Coleridge

Chapter 10
Sleep Tight

Getting the right amount of good-quality sleep is vital for good health and maintaining a healthy weight. Sleep deprivation can affect the hormones that control appetite and lead to obesity – see Chapter 2 – Eat Less. Studies show that sleeping less than five hours a night also increases the risk of heart disease, stroke, diabetes, and depression and lowers immunity. The increased risk of heart disease has been blamed on the link between too little sleep and higher levels of cortisol, the hormone linked with stress, in the bloodstream. Men who sleep poorly have been found to have lower testosterone levels, which are linked to a greater risk of developing type 2 diabetes. Insomnia can also lead to inefficiency and more time off work.

Lack of sleep can affect mood and lead to relationship problems. It can also affect co-ordination, reaction time and judgement and increase risk-taking behavior, leading to an increased risk of involvement in road or other accidents. Evidence suggests that overall, people who sleep less than six hours a night don't live as long as those who sleep seven to eight hours. Paradoxically, sleeping longer than this may also shorten the lifespan. If you sleep an average of seven to eight hours nightly and generally feel alert, you're probably getting enough sleep.

The wake/sleep cycle is governed by the circadian rhythm and the sleep homeostat. The circadian rhythm is like an internal clock, which determines when we feel like sleeping and waking. Exposure to natural light and darkness, meal times and exercise patterns can all affect it. The sleep homeostat is a mechanism controlled by brain chemicals, such as melatonin, that ensures you get enough sleep for your body to function efficiently.

If you have problems falling asleep, wake often during the night, or early in the morning, try some of these lifestyle changes to help you rebalance your wake/sleep cycle.

Make your bedroom a peaceful haven

Ensure your bed is comfortable and inviting, with fresh bedding. Buy the biggest bed you can afford, so that you or your partner can escape if one of you has a restless night. Replace a sagging mattress, or place a board between it and the base of the bed. Your pillow should keep your neck and head in line with your spine – so the most suitable height for you depends on the width of your shoulders; if you have narrow shoulders select a fairly flat pillow. If you have broad shoulders choose a deeper pillow, or use two. Make sure curtains and blinds keep the room dark – light interferes with the production of the sleep hormone melatonin. Line your curtains with blackout cloth, or invest in some blackout blinds.

QUICK T!P
SLEEP STEALERS
Don't have a TV in the bedroom, as watching TV last thing at night can overstimulate the brain and make it harder to switch off. Avoid using a computer late at night, as it can have a similar effect. The bright lights on TV and computer screens may also interfere with the hormones that regulate the sleep-wake cycle.

Keep your cool

Your brain tries to reduce your body temperature at night to slow down your metabolism. So to encourage sleep keep your bedroom fairly cool – around 16 degrees centigrade (60 degrees fahrenheit) and keep it airy.

Cotton nightwear and bedding are best for helping you to maintain a steady temperature, because cotton absorbs sweat.

If hot flashes wake you at night, sleep with a cotton sheet under the comforter (duvet). When a flush strikes, you can throw the comforter (duvet) off and still have a light cover.

Caught napping?

Some experts argue against napping during the day, claiming that it makes dropping off at night more difficult for some. However in many countries, such as Spain and Greece, taking a siesta is the norm. Recent research points to a 37 percent lower risk of a heart attack in men and women who nap for 30 minutes, at least three times a week. The results revealed even greater benefits for working men, with a 64 percent reduction in risk.

Pro-nappers claim that everyone benefits, but especially those suffering from over-tiredness and fatigue due to insufficient sleep at night. Even a 15-20 minute nap can be beneficial.

QUICK T!P

GET OUT MORE!
Research suggests that spending time outdoors during the day helps you sleep better at night. Exposure to sunlight stops the production of melatonin, making it easier for your body to produce the hormone at night, helping you to fall asleep more easily and sleep more soundly.

Enjoy exercise

Taking exercise late afternoon or early evening will increase your body temperature and metabolism, both of which will drop after about five hours, making you feel drowsy and ready to sleep. Also, research shows that people who exercise for at least half an hour four times a week sleep around 40 minutes longer than those who don't. Too little exercise can cause restlessness and problems sleeping.

Coffee curfew

Coffee contains caffeine, which acts as a stimulant. The effects can last for hours, so try not to drink coffee after 2pm. The same goes for cola. Whilst tea generally, contains less than half as much caffeine – around 50mg, it's advisable not to overdo it near bed time, if you have trouble dropping off. Alternatively, try Redbush or Rooibos tea, which is caffeine-free.

Avoid alcohol …

If you have trouble sleeping, avoid drinking alcohol near bedtime. Alcohol in general has a relaxing effect , helping you to fall asleep, but it's also a stimulant making you more likely to wake up during the night. It's also a diuretic, so you're more likely to wake up to make trips to the loo.

… but sip Sauvignon

Whilst alcohol in general is not recommended at bedtime – a glass of Cabernet Sauvignon, Merlot, or Chianti is. These wines contain grape skins that are rich in the sleep hormone melatonin.

QUICK T!P
LIMIT LIQUIDS
Generally avoid drinking large quantities of any liquid near bedtime to avoid waking to make trips to the bathroom.

No nicotine

As well as being extremely damaging to your health in general, nicotine is a stimulant, so if you must smoke, avoid smoking at bedtime. If you're using nicotine patches to help you stop smoking, be warned that they might cause vivid nightmares!

Foods that help you snooze …

Bananas are suitable for bedtime snacking because they are rich in tryptophan, the precursor to serotonin. Serotonin has a calming effect and your body uses it to produce the sleep-inducing hormone melatonin. Other foods rich in tryptophan include chicken, turkey,dairy foods, eggs, beans, rice, oats, hummus, lentils, nuts, seeds, dates,and wholegrains. A carbohydrate-rich meal increases the brain's uptake of tryptophan. Magnesium-rich foods such as seafoods, nuts, seeds, wholegrains and cooked green vegetables help to relax muscles and avoid night cramps. So an evening meal containing brown rice or pasta with chicken, or turkey and a green vegetable would help ensure a good night's sleep. A bedtime snack of nuts or seeds would also be beneficial.

… and the ones to avoid

If you have trouble dropping off, try to avoid foods that contain tyramine, an amino acid that stimulates the production of adrenaline. These include the nightshade family of vegetables i.e. potatoes, tomatoes, zucchinis (courgettes), eggplants (aubergines) and spinach. Tyramine is also found in aged or fermented foods such as beers, canned (tinned) meats, mature cheeses, salami, pepperoni and yeast extract.

Lettuce sleep

Lettuce has been recommended as a bed-time snack since Roman times. It has a sedative effect, because it contains a substance called lactucarium, which has similar properties to opium. Try adding it to a chicken or turkey sandwich.

Chilli out

Include chilli in your evening meal! Chillis contain capsaicin, which appears to help regulate the sleep cycle, allowing you to fall asleep more easily and wake up feeling more refreshed.

QUICK T!P
WRITE AWAY YOUR WORRIES
Studies suggest that stress and anxiety can disrupt sleep. If anxiety prevents you from sleeping, try writing a list of the things you need to do, or issues that are worrying you and possible solutions, before bedtime, so that you don't mull things over when you should be sleeping.

Dim the lights

Ease your body into sleep mode by reducing the level of light in the evening. This will encourage the production of the sleep hormone melatonin. A dimmer switch is ideal for this, or try winding down in lamp or candle light.

Prepare for sleep

Many of us lead increasingly hectic lifestyles that leave us unable to switch off at night, so it's important to spend an hour or two preparing for sleep. This might involve reading, watching tv, or listening to music – anything that relaxes you and helps you to 'put the day to bed'.

Bedtime ritual

Try to stick to a routine at bedtime. Follow the same ritual in the same order – for example you may take a bath first, followed by a milky drink and then read for ten minutes or so to help you wind down, before reaching for the bedside lamp. Try go to bed at the same time each night. Your body should eventually become programmed to expect sleep and release the sleep hormone melatonin as a response to following a regular routine.

Take to the tub

Take a warm bath before bed. The heat relaxes the muscles and mind. Also, sleep is normally preceded by a slight drop in body temperature which gives your body the 'message' that it's time for sleep. A warm bath raises your temperature slightly and the subsequent drop in temperature is conducive to sleep.

Enjoy a milky nightcap

A hot milky drink makes an ideal nightcap. Milk not only contains tryptophan, from which the brain produces serotonin, a hormone that makes you sleepy, it also contains calcium, which aids the process and helps you to relax. Add a vanilla pod and a little honey, for a delicious and calming bedtime drink.

Calming chamomile

Drinking chamomile tea is a well-known antidote to insomnia. It contains the amino acid glycine, which is a muscular and nerve relaxant. If you dislike the taste try adding 2 or 3 bags to a hot bath to enjoy the benefits without having to drink it!

Bedtime story

Many people find that reading in bed helps them to drop off to sleep. However, it's probably best to avoid thrillers or horror stories, as these may overstimulate the brain, making it harder to fall asleep. They may even cause nightmares!

QUICK T!P
SLEEP EASY WITH ESSENTIAL OILS
Various essential oils have calming, sedative properties. Most notably lavender, chamomile, valerian, neroli and rose. Add them to the bath, sprinkle them on your pillow, or mix with a carrier oil such as almond,

for a bedtime massage. If a stuffy nose due to cold or flu causes sleeping problems, sprinkle a few drops of eucalyptus or tea tree oil on your pillow.

Muscle relaxation

Use this technique to release tension from your muscles and aid sleep. Take a deep breath, then tense the muscles in your face. Relax and breathe out. Now work your way through your body, breathing in and out as you tense and relax each set of muscles.

Sleep regulator

To help regulate your sleep/wake cycle try a spot of DIY reflexology to stimulate your pineal gland. Using your thumb and fore-finger, massage the fleshy part about two-thirds of the way up your big toes for a one or two minutes before bedtime.

Only go to bed when you feel sleepy

Only go to bed when you feel sleepy, otherwise you may experience problems dropping off. Be aware of the difference between feeling tired and sleepy-tired. Feeling tired doesn't always mean you will be able to fall asleep, whereas feeling sleepy-tired is a sign that your body is ready for sleep. Yawning, itchy or watery eyes, having difficulty keeping your eyes open, feeling drained and aching muscles all indicate sleepiness. If you don't feel sleepy at bedtime find something to do that relaxes you, preferably away from bright lighting, until you do.

QUICK T!P

DON'T CLOCKWATCH!
If you wake during the night, try not to look at the clock, you may start worrying about how long you have left to sleep, which might prevent you from dropping off again. Instead, keep your eyes shut and try deep breathing to ease yourself back to sleep.

Get up if you can't sleep

If you don't fall asleep within what you seems like 20 minutes of going to bed or waking up during the night, get up and go into another room. You may find this hard, but it is better than tossing and turning and worrying about your lack of sleep.

Try drinking a glass of milk and doing something that you find relaxing – like reading a book, listening to soft music, or even doing a jigsaw puzzle; avoid watching TV, using the computer, or doing anything else that might overstimulate your brain.

Only go back to bed when you feel sleepy again – this will help your brain to associate your bed with sleep.

Limit the time you spend in bed

If you find yourself spending a lot of your time in bed awake, unable to sleep, try reducing the number of hours you spend there, until you begin to sleep for a higher proportion of the time. This encourages your brain to link your bed with sleep, rather than with being awake. Work out roughly how many hours you sleep each night, on average. Next, decide what time you need to get up to fit in with your work, or other commitments. For example, if you find that you usually only sleep for about six hours out of the eight you spend in bed and need to get up at 7 a.m. each morning, go to bed at 1 a.m. If you sleep less than five hours, aim to spend five hours in bed each night. Follow this schedule every night – even at weekends. Your goal is to establish a regular sleep pattern.

Finally, try to follow your natural sleep patterns – if you're a lark set your bedtime fairly early, with an early rising time; if you're an owl, go to bed later.

Jargon Buster

Amino acids	organic acids which form the building blocks of proteins.
Anti-inflammatory	reduces swelling, pain and inflammation.
Antioxidants	substances thought to neutralize free radicals.
Arteriosclerosis	narrowing of the arteries caused by fatty deposits.
Beta-carotene	the plant form of the antioxidant vitamin A, found in orange or green colored fruits and vegetables, e.g. oranges, carrots and green vegetables.
Calorie	measurement of energy in food often expressed in kcal.
Cortisol	hormone produced by the adrenal glands.
Disaccharides	sugars made up of two molecules, such as sucrose.
Diuretic	a substance that increases the amount of urine passed.
Endorphins	chemicals produced in the brain that lift mood and reduce pain.
Enzymes	proteins produced by the body which speed up biological reactions.
Flavonoids	type of polyphenol – water-soluble plant pigments that act as antioxidants.
Free radicals	cell-damaging substances produced when body burns food, or is exposed to pollution etc.

Glucosinolates	compounds found in cruciferous vegetables, such as broccoli, cabbages and Brussels sprouts. Believed to reduce cancer risk.
Glycemic index	a ranking of foods according to the effect they have on blood sugar levels.
Hesperitin	a flavonoid.
Hydrochloric acid	a component of gastric juice, a solution the stomach produces to break down food.
Insulin	hormone, secreted by the pancreas, which lowers blood sugar by directing it into the body's cells.
Inulins	carbohydrates found mainly in fruit and vegetables, that feed and stimulate the growth of existing good bacteria in the gut. Also known as prebiotics.
Isothiocyanates	produced from glucosinolates found in cruciferous vegetables and thought to reduce risk of cancer.
Lignans	plant estrogens found in cereals, fruits and vegetables.
Lutein	a natural pigment found in egg yolks, dark green leafy vegetables such as spinach, various fruits and corn.
Lycopene	a red pigment found in tomatoes and fruits such as watermelon, pink grapefruit and guava.
Lovastatin	a natural statin. Statins lower cholesterol by reducing the amount the liver produces and

	encouraging it to remove cholesterol from the bloodstream.
Macular degeneration	deterioration of part of the retina, leading to loss of vision.
Melatonin	hormone produced by the pineal gland in the brain that regulates sleep.
Metabolism	conversion of food into energy.
Monosaccharides	simple sugars, made up of one molecule, such as glucose.
Pectin	gelatin-like substance found in fruit and vegetables which provides soluble fiber.
Physiological	refers to body functions and processes.
Phytochemicals	chemicals which occur naturally in plants and are thought to be beneficial to health.
Phytonutrients	as above.
Polyphenols	compounds that provide much of the flavor, color, and taste in plants and benefit health.
Prebiotics	natural indigestible starches which feed and encourage the growth of existing good bacteria in the gut.
Precursor	a substance used by the body to produce another substance.

Quercetin	a flavonoid found mainly in onions, apples, tea and wine.
Resveratrol	a polyphenol of which grapes are a particularly good source.
Selenium	a trace mineral essential to the body.
Serotonin	a chemical involved in various bodily functions, including mood, appetite, sleep and sensory perception.
Testosterone	the main male sex hormone.
Theanine	an amino acid that has a tranquilizing effect.
Thrombosis	the formation of a blood clot in a vein or artery.
Trans-fats	formed when hydrogen is passed through unsaturated fats, to make them more solid for use in processed foods, and when oil is heated to a high temperature.
Triglyceride	the main form of fat stored in the body.
Tryptophan	amino acid that is the precursor to serotonin.
Type 2 diabetes	a condition where the body makes insufficient insulin, or the body's tissues are unable to use it effectively.
Zeaxanthin	a plant pigment found in green vegetables and yellow and orange fruits and vegetables, such as peppers, sweet corn, nectarines, oranges, papaya and butternut squash.

Index